The
POTATO
Hack

Weight Loss Simplified

BY TIM STEELE

POTATO QUOTES

"Let the sky rain potatoes!"

Falstaff in *The Merry Wives of Windsor*
William Shakespeare (1564-1616)

The information provided in this book is for your enjoyment and to provide information on the subjects discussed. This book should not be used to diagnose or treat any medical condition. For diagnosis or treatment of medical problems, consult your physician. The publisher and author are not responsible for any health or allergy problems that require medical supervision and are not liable for any damages or negative consequences from any treatment, action, application or preparation, to any person reading or following the information in this book. References and endorsements are provided for informational purposes only.

Cover Credit: Ann Overhulse Photography, Copyright © 2016

ISBN: 1530028620
ISBN-13: 978-1530028627

TABLE OF CONTENTS

Foreword(s)

"Prepare for a witty, practical, and encouraging, yet completely scientific read. *The Potato Hack* provides a valuable, all-around look at the humble, oft-shunned potato. Tim Steele leads the discussion that the potato not only belongs in your diet, but that it can also help you reclaim your health—from fighting cancer to weight optimization to recovering gastrointestinal health. Having survived my own curiosity-driven, personal three-day potato hack trial, I will vouch for its satiety factor and a 2.5 pound weight loss. Suffice it to say that the potato is proudly back on the family's table."

> — **Dr. Terri Fites, M.D.**, nutrition writer for *Molly Green Magazine*; open-minded hostess of The Homeschooling Doctor, an eclectic, personal blog devoted to exploring alternative health and alternative education in an honest, candid way; and most importantly, mother of four and head cook.

"The Potato Hack is a significant health discovery. I say this as a very conservative research biochemist. Tim had to flaunt conventional medical opinions and heal himself, before he was prepared to try a time-honored, 19th Century potato remedy. The Potato Hack is backed by recent research linking simple diets with enhanced diversity of gut microbiota, renewed immune function and improved health. It also explains how a unique soluble fiber in potatoes, resistant starch, can feed the flora and fix a lot of people. Beyond making good biochemical sense, I can vouch for the efficacy of The Potato Hack from personal experience."

> — **Dr. Art Ayers, Ph.D.**, former professor of cellular biology at Harvard University and host of Cooling Inflammation, a blog explaining the interaction of diet, inflammation and disease mediated by gut microbiota.

"This book is one of the most extensive investigations on the benefits of resistant starch around. Tim covers a large body of research surrounding his novel method of resetting the body against a whole host of ailments, from chronic inflammation, insidious weight gain, and more. He lays out the painstakingly detailed science behind the magic contained in one of our most common staples, the potato, and the biological impact resistant starch can have on the body. Definitely worth the read to get the most comprehensive rundown on the topic."

> — **Mark Sisson**, author of *The Primal Blueprint* and publisher of MarksDailyApple.com

"Sometimes the simplest approach is the best one. The Potato Hack isn't fancy, complicated, or expensive, but it's a powerful tool for weight loss."

> — **Chris Kresser**, Author of New York Times best seller *The Paleo Cure*. Creator of top-ranked natural health website ChrisKresser.com. Co-director and President of California Center for Functional Medicine

"The Potato Hack has revived the forgotten knowledge that a few days of potato-only meals might just be the ticket to resetting a sticky metabolism, losing weight, and restoring a healthy gut biome. Tim's research over the past couple years about resistant starch took the internet by storm. What was once an esoteric term, "resistant starch" is now a household word, and Paleo dieters are forever changed. Though I'm one of those genetically "gifted" people mentioned in the book whose biology is not compatible with potatoes, if you eat potatoes with impunity, the Potato Hack could be a great way to shake up a diet that has stalled, or just to push your limits the way only a true biohacker could appreciate. The Potato Hack breaks all the molds, just like Bulletproof Coffee!"

> — **Dave Asprey**, founder of Bulletproof and author of New York Times bestseller *The Bulletproof Diet*.

"Despite intermittent bad press from the media and some diet communities, potatoes have long been a staple food for healthy populations around the world, and humans have been eating tubers since Paleolithic times. I would be hard pressed to find a better single food for a short-term period of calorie restriction, which is sometimes called a 'fast' nowadays and is showing promise for weight loss and improving health markers. The fact is, the versatile potato is a nutrient dense whole food, and that's why it can also play a prominent role in *The Plant Paleo Diet* that I created for long term health, vitality, and longevity."

— **Angelo Coppola**, host and producer of the Latest in Paleo Podcast and The Plant Paleo Diet, PlantPaleo.com

Tim Steele proposed this "potato hack" as a means to rapid weight loss with good nutrition and lack of hunger. What could be better? While I'm skeptical, I always like a good self-experiment, so I put it out for others to try if they like (search 'potato hack' for many posts and hundreds of comments). Well, lots of people did try it and contrary to all sorts of 'dire warnings' from those who strictly advocate low-carb diets, most who tried it found lots of success. It lived up to the hype.

— **Richard Nikoley**, author, entrepreneur, blogger, host of FreeTheAnimal.com

Weight loss by consuming nothing but potatoes! Who would have thought it possible? It sounds incredible but it works. The Potato Hack could not have come at a better time. The World Health Organization has reported that Europe and in particular The Irish Republic, my adopted home, is heading for an obesity epidemic and the associated health issues. Tim Steele has re-invented the health benefits of the humble Potato via its resistant starch content by research and personal experimentation. Research on the benefits of prebiotic fibers, resistant starch, gut microflora diversity and short chain Fatty acids are well documented in scientific journals but has not trickled down to the general public. The Potato Hack explains how the potato can be utilized as a sole source of nutrition to enhance whole body health via feeding and modulating the composition of the gut microbiota with weight loss as a "side effect." The simplest solutions are always the best!

— **Ashwin Patel, MRPharmS, MPSI**; practicing pharmacist. Owner of websites emptyingthebowel.com and preeventacne.com.

PREFACE

I'm often asked for an "elevator speech" about the potato hack. If I had 30 seconds to explain the potato hack, I'd say:

The potato hack was modeled after a diet plan described in an 1849 medical journal. Even back then, Americans were becoming fat and "dyspeptic" [poor digestion] from eating too much. This potato diet simply called for one to eat nothing but potatoes for a few days at a time, promising that fat men become as "lean as they ought to be." 167 years later, we are fatter and sicker than ever, but the potato diet still works. Potatoes contains natural drug-like agents that affect inflammation, hunger, insulin, sleep, dreams, mood, and body weight. The potato is the best diet pill ever invented.

With that, I give you *The Potato Hack*.

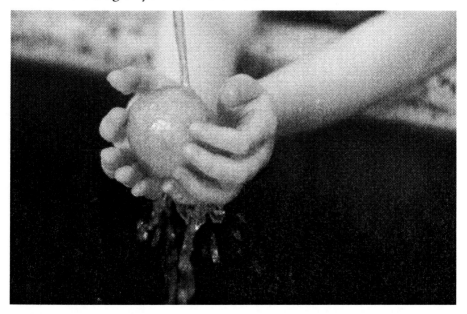

INTRODUCTION

Wouldn't it be great if you could "hack" into your body's operating system to reset the programming that stores fat and keeps you from attaining your ideal weight? Potatoes are nature's perfect weight loss and gut restoration food.

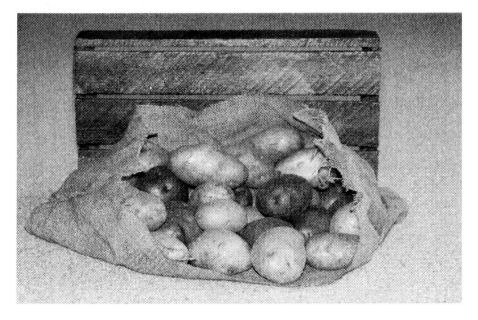

In the diet world, if it sounds too good to be true, it usually is. But the "potato hack" works. It's not a *diet*, it's a means for resetting your metabolism and restoring diversity to the trillions of bacteria that make up your gut flora. The potato hack is a short-term dietary intervention that will augment any diet plan and give you a new appreciation for your food. Along the way, most people lose 3-5 pounds after just a couple days of "potato hacking." The recipes, testimonials, and science should convince you to give it try. There is no long-term commitment required, no membership. If you don't like it, you are not out anything. Hundreds have tried the potato hack over the last 5-years and the response is overwhelming. The potato hack, as I have outlined, has been examined by doctors, scientists, nutritional experts, and researchers. All agree it's a game-changer. The potato hack works.

Who Benefits from the Potato Hack?

This book is for anyone trying to lose or maintain weight and also for anyone with digestive complaints. The potato hack works on many levels; resetting your weight set-point, increasing insulin sensitivity, flooding your system with antioxidants, and providing super nutrition to you and your gut microbiota. The potato hack restores diversity to your gut ecosystem like no probiotic pill could ever do. You can experience rapid weight loss with no hunger. Just a couple days a week and you'll be at your goal weight in no time. If you gain easily, a couple days of potato hacking per month will keep you at the weight you desire. This is truly a "hack" of epic and historical importance.

My Story

A few years ago, I was trying to lose a couple of stubborn pounds that wouldn't budge. Those dreaded "last 10" were getting the best of me. I tried low-carb, no-carb, low-calorie, no-calorie, high-fat, low-fat, high-protein—everything, or so I thought. Then I stumbled upon an article from the April 1849 edition of the *Water-cure Journal*, simply titled, "Potato Diet."

I embarked on a 14-day potato-only diet and much to my surprise, my weight, which had not budged in months, began to melt away. Within the first week I was at my goal weight of 170 pounds and by the end of the second week I weighed 164 pounds, a weight I had not seen on the scale in over 30 years.

My weight-gain journey starts in 1983. Eighteen years old and freshly out of Air Force boot camp, I had transformed from a lanky teen weighing 150 pounds into a young man weighing 165. By the end of my 6-week advanced technical training, I weighed 175 pounds. The Air Force deemed me to be within weight standards as long as I stayed under 192 pounds. Over the next 21 years, I flirted with that number many times.

Lean, Mean Fightin' Machine

One of the worst things a military person can do is become overweight. Being overweight in the military is associated with weakness and laziness. No nation wants to be represented by an army of chubby soldiers; they want "lean, mean, fightin' machines." Most branches of service have extensive "fat-boy" programs designed to teach you to eat right and exercise in a way to get your weight under control. Once in the "fat-boy" system, failure to quickly fall under your maximum allowed weight means a quick discharge and a bus ticket home to Mom and Dad. I never let myself get so overweight that I was placed on the fat-boy program, simply because I had too much at stake. I watched as many a good warrior was unceremoniously drummed out of the service because he was too fat.

My go-to trick was a week of starvation followed by two days of dehydration. I could easily lose 10 pounds by this method and as long as the scale showed less than 192 pounds, no one cared that my kidneys were screaming in pain and I had not eaten in a week. What I never really learned to do after 21 years of yo-yo dieting was to eat right. Pizza and beer were my main food groups. After turning 30, weight control became even more difficult. I tried to maintain my weight under 200 pounds and force a big loss just prior to scheduled weigh-ins. In my last couple years, I had attained the rank of E-9, Chief Master Sergeant, and was afforded the luxury of skipping mandatory weight checks. Chiefs were never on the fat-boy list, but some of us made Humpty Dumpty look skinny.

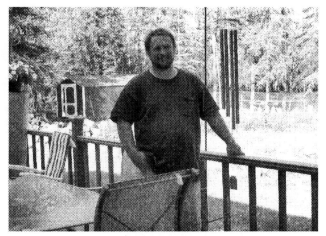

Author, 2009

Uh-oh!

When I retired from the Air Force in 2004 at age 39, I weighed on obese 210 pounds. Within 3 years, I had ballooned up to 250 pounds and developed full-fledged metabolic syndrome. I was obese with high blood pressure, high cholesterol, high triglycerides, high blood glucose (pre-diabetic), and had frequent gout attacks.

My doctor's advice to "eat less, move more, and stick to a low-fat diet" did not help me at all. It was impossible to exercise with a foot swollen from gout and I was ravenously hungry all the time. Finally, toying with different diets, I was able to start moving my weight downward. By avoiding processed foods, fried foods, sugar, and refined flour, I was able to finally get my weight under control. Soon I was off of all my medications and exercising daily.

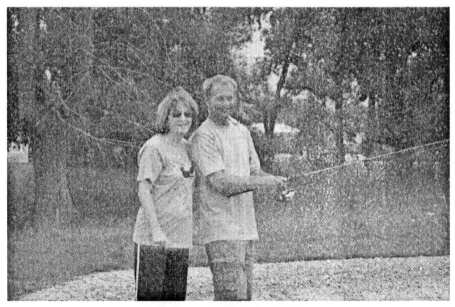

Author and wife, Jackie, 2013

Back on Track!

Early on, I had set a goal for myself of 170 pounds. It took 6-months of eating a whole-food diet to get down to 180 pounds, then the dreaded "stall" occurred. I saw 175 pounds many times, only to quickly rebound to the 180's. It was as if my body was fighting a lower weight. I had about given up on ever seeing 170 pounds when I came across the 1849 Potato Diet article. Within 2-weeks, I not only made my goal weight, but lost an additional 6-pounds. The weeks following this first "potato hack" saw even more weight loss of 3 or 4-pounds. There was no weight rebound and best of all, I felt great. This experience led me to re-evaluate everything I knew about weight loss and human health. I even returned to school for a Master's degree in biotechnology to better understand the science behind the potato hack.

How the Potato Hack Works

Just like hacking computer code, potatoes can be used to hack into the code that that keeps you lean and healthy. Not a complicated "diet," but a simple "hack," a "reset," for your metabolism. Here's a simple plan that can be used to lose weight, and keep it off, or simply to restore health to an ailing digestive system. The key component of this hack is the lowly potato. Perfectly suited to sustaining human life, the potato holds the key to resetting the way our body stores and maintains body weight by in-fluencing inflammation, set-points, and restoring key nutrients. A short-term potato-only diet has proven to be an ideal way for people to lose excess weight and keep it off, long-term. The potato hack works equally well for vegans and meat eaters, low-carb and low-fat dieters, and even for people who have never been on a diet in their entire life.

The potato hack is not just for the overweight. "Hard-gainers" who struggle trying to increase their weight and grow muscles can also benefit from this reset. Also those with a variety of gut problems such as con-stipation, diarrhea, nausea, heartburn, indigestion, can benefit from the potato hack.

> *Let those who have dyspepsia—and that means a multitude of ills which the American people in their luxurious habits are fast bringing upon themselves—try for a time the potato diet (Potato Diet, 1849).*

I'll start off by telling you about the potato hack...seven simple rules that might just end your days of worrying about weight forever. Later, we'll explore some variations and recipes. We'll also dig deep into the science behind *why* the potato hack is so effective, and how you can use other facets of potato-science to boost your immune system, gut health, and fight disease. You'll learn about something called "resistant starch" and how the potato is the world's finest source of this forgotten nutrient.

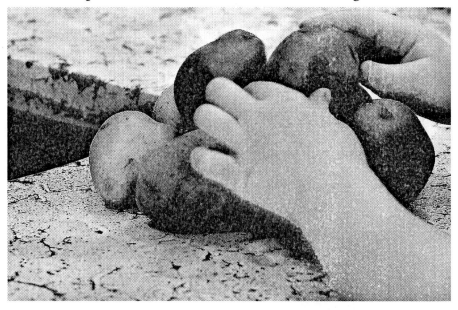

Won't People Think I'm Crazy?

Sure they will! But you'll have the last laugh. You'll need an "elevator speech" of your own to convince your friends and family that you have not gone completely mad. If you are overweight, have poor digestion, and generally of ill-health, if you are not doing something drastic to change...then maybe you *are* crazy.

Inflammation is one of the greatest threats to our health. Inflammation shows itself in subtle ways, but you can bet that if your waistline has expanded to an uncomfortable size, or you live your life by where the closest restroom is, then you undoubtedly have inflammation. Allowed to go unchecked, this inflammation will ruin your life. Inflammation and autoimmune diseases go hand-in-hand. Our "there's a pill for that" attitude is making us fatter and sicker as we get further away from the foods that can make us better. If you've tried everything, and none of it has worked for you, try the potato hack. Doctors have no pill they can prescribe that even comes close to providing the perfect blend of natural anti-inflammatory compounds found in a potato.

The Potato Reset

Originally, I was going to call this book *The Potato Reset*, but "hack" prevailed. Try the potato hack for a complete rest from your normal diet, especially if you are suffering digestion problems such as SIBO, IBS, or GERD. This is the modern, dyspeptic gut...the bane of the 21st century. Can a hack from the 19th century be the start of a new health revolution? If you've been stalled at your present weight for quite some time and you're unhappy with the diet you're on, give the potato hack a try... what have you got to lose?

> *Few are aware of the great value of the potato as an article of diet. It may astonish some of our readers when we assert that potatoes alone are sufficient to sustain the human body in a state of firm and vigorous health (Potato Diet, 1849).*

POTATO QUOTES

"WHAT I SAY IS THAT, IF A MAN REALLY LIKES POTATOES, HE MUST BE A PRETTY DECENT SORT OF FELLOW."

— A.A. MILNE (1882 – 1956)

(AUTHOR OF WINNIE-THE-POOH)

Notes:

PART 1.

WEIGHT LOSS MADE SIMPLE

CHAPTER 1. THE POTATO HACK

The rules for the potato hack are simple. If you are eating something that is not a potato, you are doing it wrong. The potato hack is for those people who gain weight easily, have a hard time losing or maintaining weight, or for anyone who wants to reset their metabolism or digestion. The potato hack is the ultimate "elimination diet."

The Rules:

1. Plan on eating *just* potatoes for 3 to 5 days
2. Eat 2-5 pounds of potatoes each day
3. No other foods allowed (this includes butter, sour cream, cheese, and bacon bits!)
4. Salt allowed, but not encouraged
5. Drink when thirsty: coffee, tea, and water only
6. Heavy exercise is discouraged; light exercise and walking are encouraged
7. Take your normal medications, but dietary supplements will not be needed

Expected results from 3-5 days of the Potato Hack:

- Fat loss of 3-5 pounds without hunger
- Reduction in inflammation and joint pain
- Reduction in digestive complaints
- Increased insulin sensitivity, lower fasting blood glucose levels
- Restoration of healthy intestinal bacteria
- Additional weight loss upon resumption of normal diet
- For weight loss, simply repeat the 3-5 day hacks weekly or every other week until you are at your goal weight

- Extra money in your pocket! The potato hack is cheap.
- An appreciation for hunger, food, and the knowledge that you can change your metabolism

---

Our word for it, the experiment will prove a good one; and the prescription costs no money, but, what is incomparably better, an amount of self-denial which is possessed only by a few (Potato Diet, 1849).

Many of us have a tendency to gain weight as we get older and most of us gain weight in the winter. The trouble with "winter weight" is that it does not magically melt in the spring like the snowman in your yard. The National Institutes of Health describe this as *unintentional weight gain*, or "weight that you gain without trying to do so when you are not eating or drinking more." They attribute this unintentional weight gain mostly to an aging metabolism, hormones, and drugs. Emotional stress, cessation of smoking, or working night shifts can also cause unintentional weight gain. A periodic potato hack can erase this unintentional weight gain. More about weight maintenance and long-term diets later!

After a couple days of potato hacking, many people report that, for the first time in years, they are not hungry. People report better sleep and habitual snorers *stop snoring*. Those that have watched an un-budging scale for months or years report daily losses of ½ to 1 pound, and the weight does not come back on, as in other "crash" diets.

The most incredible aspect of the potato diet is not the erasure of pounds or the disappearance of an achy joint but the new appreciation of the foods you take for granted in your normal diet. Your taste buds will feel alive. You will appreciate every morsel you put into your mouth. You will finally understand the phrase, "Eat to live, don't live to eat!"

> *We have tried it not for months, but a few days at a time—long enough to satisfy us of its good effects; long enough, too, to teach us well how good bread and apples and peaches are. We are far from believing that God created wheat, rye, corn, barley, buckwheat, etc.; chestnuts, beechnuts, butternuts, walnuts, etc., etc.; apples, pears, peaches, plums, grapes, and ten thousand other delicious things, not to be eaten by man (Potato Diet, 1849).*

What I have seen personally, and in the many hundreds whom I've convinced to give the potato hack a try, is that eating in this fashion will cause rapid fat loss with no loss of muscle tone or dehydration. Losses of 1 pound per day are common. Sustained weight loss of 3-4 pounds per week is commonly reported from people who have been unable to lose weight by any other means or who have been stalled in a weight loss plateau for months. The human body is an amazing piece of machinery and is fully capable of extracting all the nutrition it needs from the humble potato. So whether you need to lose 5 pounds or 100, give the potato hack a try. You'll love the 3-5 day increments…and you'll love the results.

> *Lean men grow fat, and fat men become lean—lean as they ought to be. And so all grow better in health. (Potato Diet, 1849).*

The Potato Hack Decoded

The seven easy rules I've outlined for the potato hack look simple enough. If you are eating something that is not a potato, you are doing it wrong. Yet, I've answered thousands upon thousands of questions over the past five years on exactly *how* to eat nothing but potatoes. Let's get down and dirty and dig into the potato hack, line-by-line.

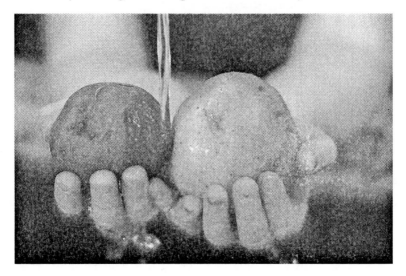

Potato Hack Rule #1: Plan on eating just potatoes for 3 to 5 days

Sounds easy enough, until around noon on Day 2, when you realize that you are almost out of potatoes, and the potatoes you do have, are not cooked. Or, on Day 3, when the guys at work decide to order pizza and you look woefully at your Ziplock baggy full of cold, boiled spuds...

This is the hardest rule for people to comprehend and adhere to. The potatoes you choose can be from the supermarket, farm stand, or your own garden. They don't have to be organic, but certainly can be. These potatoes need to be white potatoes, sometimes called Irish potatoes, and not sweet potatoes. Potatoes come in many different varieties—there are Russets, reds, yellows, whites, and blues. All are equally fine, but your preferred cooking method and time of year may dictate which variety you prefer. Sweet potatoes are not allowed because they are a completely different plant species with a completely different nutritional makeup.

> *And yet, as before said, we advise our dyspeptic friends to make a trial of the potato diet…Our word for it, the experiment will prove a good one. And making this experiment for one week will greatly increase the self-denial and perseverance of those who go through with it (Potato Diet, 1849).*

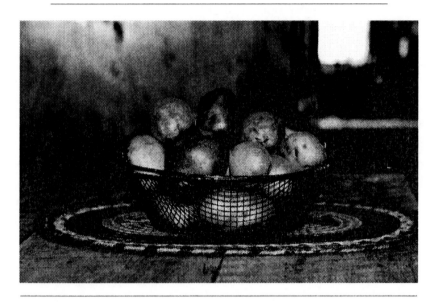

So Many Potatoes!

There are 4 types of "white" potato (Solanum tuberosum):

White – *Russet type potato, high starch content, best for baking.*

Yellow – *Yukon Gold type potato, medium starch, all-around general uses.*

Red – *Round and red, best for boiling, roasting, and potato salad.*

Blue – *Small and blue, not very common, medium starch, general use.*

Sweet Potatoes (Ipomoea batatas) and yams (Dioscorea) are <u>not</u> white potatoes.

Rule #1 has three components: planning, potatoes, and time. Your only source of nutrition should be from potatoes. We'll discuss "allowable extras" in rules 3, 4, and 5. But the #1 rule of potato hacking is: Eat Only Potatoes.

Now, you could do the potato hack for weeks at a time if you wanted. I did it for 14 days the first time I tried, lost about 10 or 12 pounds. I don't think there is much danger in doing this, but I worry about long term nutrient deficiencies with such prolonged eating of just potatoes. As we'll see later in the book, lots of people throughout history have proven that potatoes can sustain humans for months or years, but in this case, we are a bunch of humans who've become overweight for whatever reason, and may not be in peak physical shape.

Three days is so easy to do it's ridiculous. Five days gets a bit tedious. When you start talking 7+ days, you get into the weekend and it starts to fall apart. But here's the best part...the fat loss starts on day 1 and continues as long as you eat just potatoes, there is no acclimation required, and no "starvation-mode" plateau. Losing extra fat and maintaining your weight is a lifelong "hack." Using 3-5 days of potato hacking once a week to lose weight, then once a month, or a couple times a year, to maintain your weight is much easier to do than stressing your body with extended dieting of any type.

Planning is paramount. Make sure you buy enough potatoes, and pre-cook about half of them so that you always have some ready-to-eat potatoes on hand. Don't start a potato hack the day before your office Christmas party, and don't plan a potato hack when you have company coming to stay with you. A great plan is a Monday through Wednesday or Monday through Friday hack.

Three to five days seems to be the sweet-spot for meaningful weight loss. Done weekly, you can easily lose 10 pounds per month. [For the die-hard dieters out there, you know *that's huge*!] Done monthly, you can easily keep your weight in-check year 'round without being overly mindful of what you eat. I will say, though, your normal diet probably needs some tweaking if you have trouble maintaining your weight. We'll talk about that later.

To recap, rule #1 is about the food and the time it takes to pull off a successful Potato Hack. A bit of planning will go a long, long way it making your first hack a success.

Potato Hack Rule #2: Eat 2-5 pounds of potatoes each day

The key to success with the potato hack is proper planning. Nothing can be worse than running out of potatoes on the second day, and since you don't know exactly how many potatoes you will need to eat, this is a distinct possibility. If you are a human being who weighs between 100 and 300 pounds, then for planning purposes figure on eating three pounds of potatoes a day. You may have some left over, or you may need more, but this figure seems to hold true for everyone to achieve a level of fullness and see amazing weight loss.

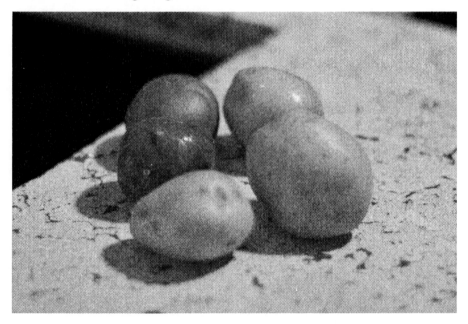

If you want to jump right in to a 5-day potato hack, then you'll need to buy 15-20 pounds of potatoes. I like to get some extra since you may find a couple bad ones or a couple that have bad spots that you need to trim. Try to purchase potatoes that are equally sized, roughly the size of a tennis ball or baseball. Weigh them at the store—they should go about 2 or 3 to the pound. You don't want giant potatoes, they are hard to cook—and you don't want tiny potatoes, they are hard to peel. Look closely at the potatoes you buy. Ensure there are no excessive eyes, or sprouts, growing on them. Make sure they are not moldy or rotten. Look for indications of greening. You need to get the best quality potatoes you can find. Eventually you will get the hang of selecting your potatoes and it will be easier each time.

When you arrive home with your bounty of spuds, the first thing you should do is wash and peel 10-15 of them. Ensure there are no black or green spots. Some of this can be trimmed away, but if they don't look appetizing, don't eat them. You may wish to cut the potatoes into quarters or halves to check the insides for hollowing or black spots—throw those away.

Now you are ready to cook your first batch. I recommend you boil them in a pot of lightly salted water. Bring to a boil and simmer 10-15 minutes until the potatoes are tender, but not falling apart. You want a center that is still very firm, if not uncooked. When the potatoes are done, drain them well and allow to cool. If you want to eat some right way, dig in. Store the rest in a suitable container in your refrigerator until you are ready to eat them. Use these as your emergency stock, snacks, and for lunches. There is nothing more filling than munching on a cold potato when hunger calls your name. These cold potatoes can also be quickly reheated in the microwave or cubed and heated in a non-stick pan for quite delicious home-fries. See the recipes section for more cooking ideas.

For the sake of safety, I recommend peeling supermarket potatoes. Some people prefer to peel all of their potatoes; that's fine, too. Potatoes contain solanine, a compound found in the leaves, shoots, and sometimes skin of potatoes. Solanine in high concentrations can cause illness and discomfort in everyone, and some people are more sensitive than others. Since you will be eating more potatoes than you ever have in your entire life, please take the time to carefully inspect each potato.

If you grow your own potatoes, or buy local, organic, you still need to inspect each potato for signs of greening or sprouting. I realize I shouldn't have to tell you this, as you've all eaten potatoes your entire lives without a problem, but there are many people who simply do not normally buy or eat real potatoes.

Later on, we'll discuss the nutrition of the potato, but for the sake of rule #2, a pound of potatoes contains 350 calories (79 grams carbs, 11 grams protein, and .5 grams fat). Our 2-5 pound rule will allow you to eat between 700-1800 calories per day, with 160-400g of carbs, 22-55g of protein, and even a couple grams of fat. Calorie counters will recognize this break down, most diets try to emulate what the potato provides naturally.

Lastly, don't sweat the exact weight of the potatoes you are eating. Weights are all "as purchased." And never, ever set a goal for a certain number of potatoes to eat. Eat until full and stop.

To recap, rule #2 says to eat 2-5 pounds of potatoes a day, this will provide all of the calories, energy, and nutrients you need to survive without feeling starved. The goal of the Potato Hack is not to eat as many potatoes as you can, but just enough potatoes to get you through the day.

Potato Hack Rule #3: No other foods allowed

You'd think this would go without saying. No one wants to believe the potato hack *really* means *just* potatoes. Surely an apple or a cheeseburger won't interfere, right? Wrong! A big part of the magic of the potato hack is the singularity of food. When you present your taste buds with all manner of goodies, your brain demands more. Hunger signals tell your 4 million-year-old food acquisition system to go out and seek more of these tasty treats. And you willingly obey.

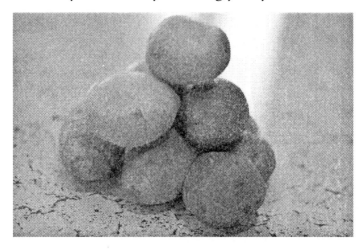

Let's dissect the primary rule, "Eat Potatoes Only." These three simple words seem to be incomprehensible to most people. Hardly anyone alive today has ever eaten *potatoes only* for any length of time. Many people have never even eaten a *plain* potato.

For the purpose of rule #3, "other foods" are considered caloric, nutritional food and drink.

- Breakfast smoothie? No!
- Mid-morning power-bar? Gone!
- Afternoon ice cream? Absolutely not!
- Need a suitable replacement? Potato, potato, potato.

Get it? No other foods allowed.

But let's face it. What's a potato without butter, sour cream, chives, and bacon bits? Potatoes are supposed to be *fully loaded*. Mashed potatoes are nothing without gravy. French fries are nothing if not soaked in trans-fat cooking oil and slathered in ketchup. Hash browns gotta be soaked in truck stop grease and covered in Tabasco. Plain, you say? Craziness!

Rule #3 also includes toppings. There are many ways to prepare potatoes that don't require a ton of toppings. Boiled, baked, roasted, fried, or mashed…all of these taste wonderful…when you are *hongry*. That's right, *hongry*. A step past hungry.

Remember when people used to say, "Eat only when hungry?" Well, with the potato hack, you will definitely learn what this means. Not many people go hungry, let alone *hongry*, in 2016. Trust me, if you are not hungry enough to eat a plain, cold boiled potato, you ain't *hongry*.

To recap, rule #3 says: Eat. Only. Potatoes. Got it? Good.

Potato Hack Rule #4: Salt is OK

I've been guiding people through potato hacks longer than anyone. As much as I hate to see it, I can understand why people feel the need to dress their spuds up a bit. Salt is hard-wired into our brains as a "required" flavor, this is for a reason. We need to consume sodium. It helps control bodily fluids and muscle contractions among other things. Too little salt can be just as bad as too much. Luckily our cravings for salt are generally just right to keep us supplied with sodium. Potatoes contain sodium. Three pounds of potatoes contain about 75mg of sodium. If you normally salt your foods or if you find yourself craving salt, feel free to sprinkle some on your spuds.

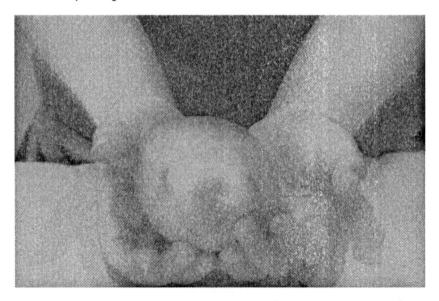

The original 1849 diet calls for just plain potatoes and I believe there is merit to sticking with that concept. It is just human nature to want to tweak everything to suit your desires. I know first-hand that as soon as I start adding in spices and bits of other food, it stops being the potato hack and starts just being a calorie-restricted diet where I'm hungry all the time.

> *Eat, of course, no salt, no butter, or condiments of any kind. (Potato Diet, 1849).*

There is a beautiful simplicity to eating only potatoes once you've convinced yourself it is safe to do so. It's almost as if your brain just gives up on making you seek out new food sources. When you resolve to eat *only potatoes* for a set length of time, it's almost as if your brain stops its incessant cries for you to eat, eat, eat.

I'd like to offer a challenge. Your very first potato hack should include a day or two of nothing but plain potatoes. This will earn you "bragging rights" if nothing else, and let you see what it's like to truly be on the potato diet as described in 1849.

To recap, rule #4 says: Salt…meh. If you absolutely must. But try without.

Potato Hack Rule #5: Drink when thirsty...coffee, tea, water

If you are a consummate coffee drinker like me, you will appreciate this rule. Otherwise, just drink water when you are thirsty. Potatoes are watery on their own, but don't let yourself get dehydrated. Coffee and tea are full of wonderful chemicals that aid almost any fat loss efforts, even decaf. If you are not a coffee and tea drinker, you might even think about starting.

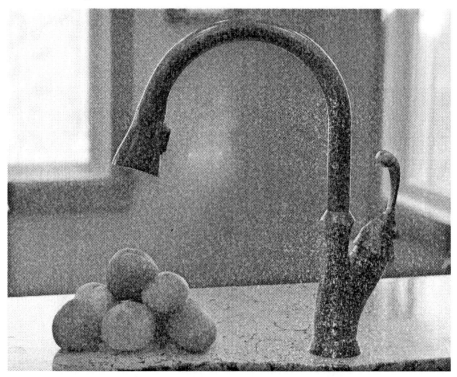

Now let's talk about that sugar and cream. It will be tough, but you are going to have to give it up or cut waaaaay back. Use Stevia instead of sugar, if you must "lighten" your coffee, do it with low fat milk, not heavy cream. Don't even think about putting a stick of butter in your coffee, please. Never heard of buttered coffee? People *do* that. It's a *thing*. Google it.

Here's a little hint on the uniqueness of the potato hack: all the diets that promise rapid weight loss do so by dehydration. If you fast for 24 hours, you'll almost certainly lose 5 or 6 pounds, but upon resumption of normal eating, you'll gain it all back. Extreme low carb diets deplete your body of "glycogen." Your body converts carbs to glycogen and stores it in your muscles and liver, mainly. Each pound of glycogen absorbs three or four pounds of water, so getting rid of dietary carbs also gets rid of glycogen and water. People on low carb diets eating off-plan very often gain 5-10 pounds seemingly overnight.

For now, just ensure you drink plenty of fluids. Off-limits are calorie-containing drinks, i.e. sports drinks, soda-pop, fruit juice. In fact, while we're at it, if you drink this stuff normally…stop. You drink water, you eat food. Don't drink your food! I know smoothies are all the rage, but treat them like food, not water.

To recap, rule #5 says: Stay hydrated. Drink plenty of water. Coffee and tea are fine, but lay off the cream and sugar.

Potato Hack Rule #6: Exercise

Bodybuilders figured this one out a long time ago. As Jack LaLanne said, "Exercise is king. Nutrition is queen. Put them together and you've got a kingdom." Bodybuilders are very aware of body fat. "If it jiggles, it's fat," as Arnold Schwarzenegger likes to say. These guys all know the deal. Building muscle and losing fat are two ends of a spectrum and are not done simultaneously. Bulking and cutting, as it's known, means eating and exercising like there's no tomorrow, then dieting furiously. In the process, they get a bit "jiggly." Just before a competition, they cease all heavy exercise and stop eating so much. This removes the excess fat and gives them that lean, "ripped" look.

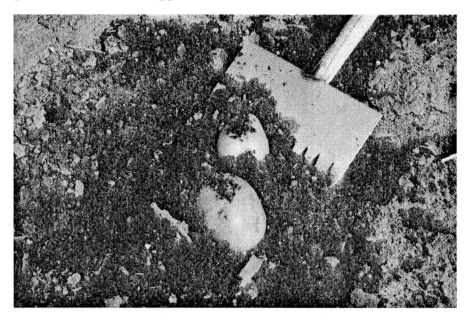

> *We do not, of course, recommend this prescription to those who have to labor very hard, for a sudden change, of whatever kind, does not answer well with such (Potato Diet, 1849).*

Pumping iron is not a fat-burning exercise. Light jogging and some easy exercises like pushups, squats, and planks are good fat-burning exercises. Walking trumps them all, however. Walking puts you squarely in the "fat-burning" zone. Personally, I think everyone should walk at least 30 minutes a day, even if broken into three, 10-minute walks. Everyone who exercises benefits from periodic rest days. This feature is present in every strenuous exercise program from CrossFit to P90X. Even the Jillian Michaels "30 Day Shred" program has one rest day per week, and Jillian *never* rests! So, use the potato hack as your rest days if you are a big exerciser. Guaranteed you will not lose all your hard-earned muscle. In fact, potatoes contain a chemical called "chlorogenic acid" which may help increase your muscles without even trying. Bodybuilders know chlorogenic acid as a secret weapon for building huge muscles, but few realize it's found naturally in potatoes.

To recap, rule #6 says: Keep calm and eat potatoes.

Potato Hack Rule #7: Medications and dietary supplements

I guess this is the point where I should be adding in a standard disclaimer for you to "check with your physician before starting the potato hack." But I won't do that. The FDA does not regulate the medicinal effects of real food. Potatoes, being real food, are not considered medicine. However, if you are taking proton pump inhibitors (PPIs) for heartburn, IBS, or GERD, you will undoubtedly find that on day 2 of the potato hack, you no longer need your meds. If you are taking pain killers or anti-inflammatory drugs for arthritis pain, you may also find that on Day 2 you don't need your daily fix.

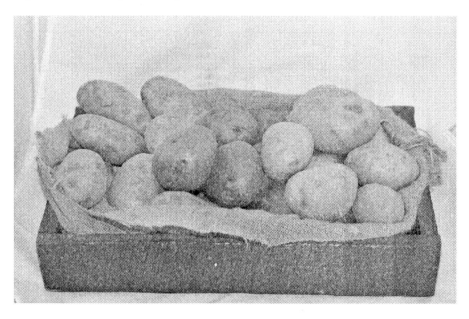

More than one person has told me over the years that they do periodic potato hacks just for the relief of arthritis pain. Others have told me they do it just so they can lower their fasting blood glucose (FBG) levels. Others have said, "Wow, my libido!" Later in the book we'll discuss the potato's pharmacologic properties. I think you'll be surprised to read exactly how medicinal potatoes really are.

> *Strange enough is it that the potato diet cures almost all who are subjected to its influence a few months (Potato Diet, 1849).*

Supplements. The dieting world is enamored with dietary supplements. Vitamins, minerals, and every sort of nutritional aid are for sale everywhere we look. The supplement industry is worth billions of dollars, rivaling the profits of Big Pharma. Is the food we eat so devoid of nutrition that we must receive nourishment from a pill bottle? I'm here to tell you that many of your health problems are *compounded* by all of the excess vitamins and minerals you take. Even much of our food is fortified with vitamins and minerals we wouldn't need if we just ate real food.

To recap, rule #7 says: Take your meds, but drop the supplements while potato hacking.

POTATO QUOTES

"SMEAGOL WON'T GRUB FOR ROOTS AND CARROTSES AND - TATERS. WHAT'S TATERS, PRECIOUS, EH, WHAT'S TATERS?"

"PO-TA-TOES!" SAID SAM."

— J.R.R. TOLKIEN, THE TWO TOWERS

Notes:

Chapter 2. Variations on the Basic Hack

The seven rules of the potato hack work extremely well as written. The first time you try the potato hack, please follow it closely. Once you've done a round, evaluate how it worked. Did you see any weight loss or other benefits? There is no disgrace in hating the potato hack. Admittedly, it's not for everyone. That's where these variations come in.

Over the years, as people try to bribe and coerce me into allowing other foods on the "potato" hack, there have been some unique variations proposed. I've personally tried all of these. Some work great, some not so great *for me*. Some folks swear by their favorite variation. These variations take into account the unique nature of the human being, our need for control, and a desire to continually tweak everything we do. Consider these variations as "hacking the hack." You may even come up with your own hack.

Spice it up

I believe the potato hack derives much of its power from blandness. There is no "party in your mouth" when you are eating potatoes, although, as you'll see, plain potatoes can be very tasty. Salt is allowed in the basic version of the hack. I don't know of anyone who found the potato hack did not work as advertised simply due to the extra salt. If anything, salt makes it work a bit better at reducing inflammation and burning fat. Therefore, the first variation I'll describe is a spiced-up version of the 1849 potato hack.

The spices used in this variation are the typical dried spices you'd normally cook with. Fresh and organic spices are a plus. A sprinkle of seasoned salt makes potatoes much more enjoyable but there are a couple of spices that go extremely well with potatoes. Black pepper, paprika, and rosemary are the accoutrement of choice by professional chefs. If you'd like to take a trip down memory lane (way, way down) in the Andes Mountains where potatoes originated, you'll find a couple of spices native to the region that were most certainly used on potatoes. Cilantro, mint, oregano, and hot pepper are all native to the area where potatoes were first eaten.

Though not technically spices, lemon juice and vinegar also make potatoes very flavorful without adding calorically to the meal. Vinegar also has a great quality that, when added to a starchy meal, it will reduce the glucose spike. Dieters have long been told to add vinegar to starchy meals. Vinegar and potatoes are a unique flavor combination popular in different parts of the world. Some swear by salt and vinegar for potatoes, anything else being overkill.

My only qualm with "spicing it up" is that I feel it's cheating. Please, get to know the potato first. Try it plain, for a full day at least. People who have told me that potatoes "suck" are quite surprised when they first try a Yukon Gold or a German Butterball. Most potatoes are tasty. The big brown baking potatoes you find in the supermarket are not known for flavor. Try out some other varieties, make a game of it, you will not regret it.

Summary: Try a variety of spices on your potatoes while potato hacking. Bonus points if you use fresh, organic spices. <u>Do not</u>, under any circumstance, use artificial flavors (bacon, lemon, etc…) these are not spices, just chemicals. For best results use:

- Black Pepper
- Paprika
- Rosemary
- Cilantro
- Oregano
- Mint
- Basil
- Cayenne Pepper
- Garlic
- Onion
- Fresh Lemon Juice

Potatoes by Day

This is quite possibly my favorite variation. It's a riff on Mark Bittman's *Vegan Before 6:00* (VB6) diet plan. "Potatoes by Day" or "PBD" is just as it sounds, from sunup 'til sundown, you just eat potatoes. In other words, potatoes for breakfast, lunch, and snacks and then a dinner of whatever you'd like.

Nutrition-wise, PBD is much easier than VB6. The VB6 book has an extensive collection of recipes, unlike The Potato Hack. Eating a great vegan diet is hard to do, which is why Bittman allows a normal dinner. Unless the practitioners of vegan diets do some reading, they can fall into vegan traps which make a vegan diet possibly worse than a diet of fast food and candy. For instance, let's say your version of VB6, or any vegan diet, involves a vegan muffin for breakfast, made with trans fats and high fructose corn syrup. Then lunch is a trip to McDonald's where you pick up a small salad and a large order of fries. Add a couple power bars or Reese's Peanut Butter Cups for snacks. Vegan for sure, but healthy? Not on your life.

> Furthermore, I had no interest in becoming an isolated vegan in a world of omnivores…(Bittman, *Vegan Before 6:00*, 2013).

PBD takes away the uncertainty of an unhealthy vegan diet. There are no choices, other than to use salt or not. Many people, including me, simply do not do well in a world of plenty. Maybe our ancestors were constantly starved and the lucky off-spring who continually sought food survived. Potatoes by Day takes away the choices and bad decisions you make; and it's highly nutritious. Some Irish peasants survived their entire life on a diet of oatmeal, potatoes, and milk. These three foods led to a population explosion and one of the healthiest populations the world had seen. Just imagine how healthy our world would be today if everyone ate potatoes from morning 'til night and a well-balanced dinner.

Try PBD for your maintenance diet. There is absolutely no harm in doing PBD literally forever. If your dinner has a bit of meat, some whole grains, and fruit and vegetables you will be the most well-nourished kid on your block. Vegan diets have merit, for sure, but also shortfalls. Most vegans take a vitamin B12 supplement because this vital nutrient cannot be had from plants. With PBD, you will not need any supplements. The potatoes will be your multi-vitamin and a "normal" dinner removes any food restrictions that could lead to malnutrition.

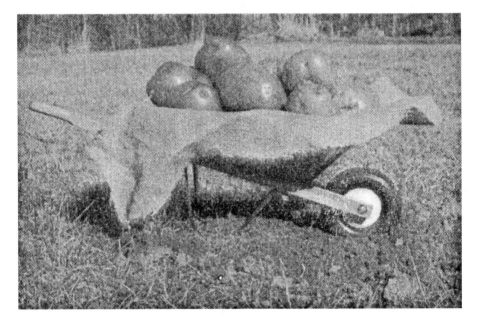

If you are a vegan and find yourself overweight, PBD may be just what you need. The Potatoes by Day variation lends itself nicely to many variations of its own. You can try PBD during the work week, on weekends, or for a week or month at any time of your choosing. I think you'll find you will never get tired of the tasty potato dishes in the recipe section, and eating this way makes dinner oh-so-much more enjoyable. Try PBD for a week. You'll love it.

Summary: Potatoes by Day, or PBD, is a simple method of increasing your potato intake to meaningful levels. The "hack" remains intact though you eat a normal dinner. While PBDing, try to be as "1849" as you can, don't combine PBD with variations. Dig deep into your willpower and eat only plain potatoes by day. If it works well, then experiment with the variations to make it just a bit easier. Your potato intake on PBD will be about 1-2 pounds per day.

Potato "PUDDD"ing

This is a spin-off of Johnson UpDayDownDay Diet™. Often abbreviated JUDDD™, this diet is one of the trademarked low carb diets that seems to work exceptionally well for people who enjoy a low carb approach to dieting. With JUDDD™, one has days of high calories and days of low calories. The book associated with JUDDD™ is *The Alternate Day Diet* which promises activation of your "skinny gene." If you are shopping for a diet plan, take a look, maybe you'll like it. The *Alternate Day Diet* is filled with many of the same "alphabet soup" strategies for success that I use here in *The Potato Hack*.

> *The Alternate-Day Diet* is based on scientific and clinical studies that show how restricting calories only every other day activates a gene called SIRT1, the skinny gene.

With PUDDD, simply eat your normal diet one day, and potato hack the next. With JUDDD™, you'll need to go through an extensive "induction" period and use a series of calculations to determine your basal metabolic needs for your down days. The down days of JUDDD™ are simply calorie reduced days and the up days are eating normally. The danger of this diet is that the user may never really learn to eat properly and simply switch between starving and eating crappy food. With PUDDD, the same trap is there…you'll need to learn to eat right on your up days. However, the down days of PUDDD are so easy, even a caveman could do it (sorry, Paleo®). Just eat potatoes until you are full on your down days. No counting calories, no tracking nutrients. The potato is the ideal food for an "up day, down day" approach to eating.

PUDDD would be great for a long term maintenance plan, or for slow, sustained weight loss. For maintenance, try PUDDD for a week at a time, once every month or even just a couple times a year. For weight loss, try PUDDD for a month and see what happens. The weight loss will be undoubtedly slower than straight potato hacking, but PUDDD shows great promise in keeping people on track. With PUDDD, you can use any of the other variations here on your potato down day. You'll be able to see what works and switch things up to keep it interesting.

I can't stress enough that you will need to learn to eat a human-appropriate diet. This is as simple as just avoiding the big 3 industrial foods: Refined sugar, industrially processed oil, and enriched wheat. If a food label lists any of those as the main ingredients, don't eat it. Ever.

Summary: PUDDD involves alternate day dieting. Every other day, do a potato hack. After a short while, you will see a downward trend in your weight. PUDDD works particularly well around the holidays where food-based gatherings are frequent.

Added Oil or Fat

For some strange reason, the first thing people want to do on an all-potato diet is to cook them in fat. I'm really not a fan of this variation, and I've scratched it off the list several times only to add it back when I ruin yet another frying pan. Using some type of fat does making cooking much easier and imparts a bit of crispy mouthfeel.

What kind and how much? This is the million-dollar question. I've experimented with coconut and olive oil with good success. I'd suggest that if you need to use some oil, stay completely away from the industrial seed oils of corn, Canola, peanut, and the so-called vegetable oils. Margarine is not a real food and should be avoided. My list of possible potato hack oils is fairly short:

- Coconut oil
- Palm oil
- Olive oil
- Butter
- Ghee
- Animal fat ("drippings," grease, lard, etc..)

These are the only cooking fats I recommend for anyone, ever, but if you want to use a different one, it's up to you. As to a proper amount, let's say about 1 teaspoon (tsp) per pan. A teaspoon of oil weighs 4.5 grams and has about 40 calories. It does not take much oil to place it in the majority of calories for a meal. To make your oil go further, use a spray type oil, but please stay away from the pressurized "cooking sprays" that are so popular. Read the ingredients and if you see dimethylpolysiloxane, diacetyl, and any type of propellants, do not use. This goes for always, not just potato hacking. Consider that my public service announcement.

The proper amount of oil to use is not measured in teaspoons or grams, it's the amount that is *juuuust* enough to allow you to cook a particular potato dish that requires a bit of oil to prevent sticking. The perfect amount is none. If you find that you need a ton of oil with every meal, maybe it's time for some self-reflection. Parchment paper can be used in place of oil in any dish that is baked.

The low-fat aspect of the potato diet is one of the keys to its success. This is an extreme low fat diet, not just a "lite" diet. When you start adding fats to your meals, the entire physiology of the meal changes. During the potato hack, every single drop of fat your body needs to fuel itself should come from body fat, not food. Your body needs fat, that's why it stores it on your thighs and belly. Let's make our body work for its fat for a change.

Summary: Try adding a bit of oil, but only to aid in cooking. If you are eating more than a small spoonful of oil daily while potato hacking, you likely will not see the results you had hoped for.

Meat & Potatoes

We've all heard folks described as "meat and potatoes" people. Maybe they are onto something. To succeed with the Meat & Potatoes hack, you must keep your meat portion small and lean. You'll also find that a long separation between eating the meat and your all-potato meal will add to the success.

For instance, have an all-potato breakfast of something like oven-baked curly fries, oil-less hash browns, or a plain boiled potato. For lunch, a half of a lean chicken breast or a piece of baked cod. Try to keep it to around 4 ounces, or the size of a deck of cards. Some people seem to really need meat in their diet and a small piece helps keep them on track. Maybe you'd rather have the meat at breakfast or dinner. No problem. Just don't get in the habit of having a big potato meal, and then scarfing down a pack of bacon. It won't work.

Summary: A small piece of lean meat, eaten several hours before your normal potato meals, seems to not interfere with potato hacking. Your mileage may vary!

Potatoes and Gravy

If there ever was a more natural pair, I don't know what. Potatoes and gravy just *go* together. In this variation, we pair potatoes with a very benign ingredient, broth. Broth, be it chicken broth, "bone" broth, or simply a stock made of vegetables, is very healthy. It's hardly food, more a drink. Little more than water and some nutrients, it can be quite flavorful but with hardly any calories, especially when all traces of fat are skimmed from the top. My nutrition calculator shows chicken broth has only 20 calories per cup. That's quite a deal.

Here's the best part: what is more "potato" than potato starch? Potato starch's #1 use is in the making of gravy.

Here's the recipe:

- 2 cups of chicken broth
- 1 Tablespoon of potato starch

Instructions: Pour ½ cup of cold chicken broth in a small bowl and set aside. Bring the rest of the chicken broth to a slow boil. While the broth is heating up, add 1TBS of potato starch to the cold broth in the bowl and stir vigorously. When the broth in the pan is boiling, slowly add the starch/broth mixture while stirring. Within seconds the potato starch will gelatinize and become a perfectly thickened gravy that can be used as a sauce on any potato dish.

Yep, that's it. Two ingredients. Makes enough to last nearly a week. You don't need much of this wonderful gravy to moisten your spuds. A bit of salt and pepper and you won't even know this is the potato hack, for good or bad. Not that I want to rain on your parade, but don't make the potato hack *too* easy. As Scrooge said to Marley's ghost:

> You may be an undigested bit of beef, a blot of mustard, a crumb of cheese, a fragment of underdone potato. There's more of gravy than of grave about you, whatever you are! (Charles Dickens, *A Christmas Carol*, 1843).

Summary: Try your hand at making homemade gravy using potato starch and broth. You'll probably carry this recipe over into everyday life, *it's that good.*

Ipomoea batatas Hack

Ipomoea batatas is better known as "sweet potato." For the purpose of this variation, we'll also throw in yams since most people can't tell them apart and they are often mislabeled at the store. The nutritional profile of sweet potatoes, yams, and white potatoes is different. Sweet potatoes have much less starch and more sugar.

Below we have the nutrition profiles for three pounds of white potato and a comparable amount of sweet potato. While the nutritional differences may not seem like much, each has its own unique signature. I've talked with several people who have successfully used sweet potatoes or yams as a portion of their potatoes on the potato hack, though I cannot personally vouch for the effectiveness or the satiety of yams and sweet potatoes. This variation has not been well-tested and it is a completely different hack, if it works.

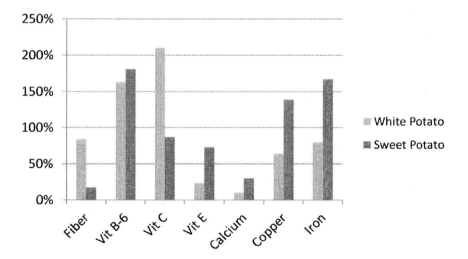

Sweet Potato vs White Potato (% of RDA)

This variation is my least favorite, but you might like it. Simply substituting a couple sweet potatoes in a meal, or having a couple sweet potato/yam meals will most likely not be problematic. For people with nightshade sensitivities, this may be the hack for you. Sweet potatoes and yams are not from the nightshade family and do not have the solanine and chaconine that causes problems for some people with white potatoes.

Summary: If you cannot tolerate regular potatoes, try sweet potatoes or yams. For variety on a potato hack, an added sweet potato or yam should be well-tolerated.

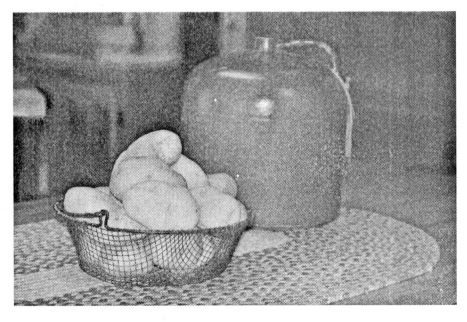

Conclusion

The variations are endless but I'm quite pleased with these. You could even mix and match, for instance, meat & potatoes fried in a bit of oil with spices and gravy. Is that taking it too far? It's a "legal" combination but you'll have to decide. The intent of these variations is not to create a way to eat even more potatoes, but to break up the monotony and possible unpalatability of potatoes in the hands of amateur cooks. Try hard, dig deep. I'd rather hear that these variations are not needed, or possibly, that they helped you stick to a mostly true potato hack.

POTATO QUOTES

"FOR ME, A PLAIN BAKED POTATO IS THE MOST DELICIOUS ONE....IT IS SOOTHING AND ENOUGH."

M.F.K. FISHER (1908 – 1992)

PREEMINENT AMERICAN FOOD WRITER

Notes:

Chapter 3. Weight Loss and Maintenance Strategies

The potato hack has undeniable physiological effects on the overweight body. We can use these effects to lose and maintain weight effortlessly. Weight loss is normally achieved through some strict calorie counting scheme or manipulating the macronutrients (protein, fat, carb) to force a calorie deficit. Weight loss without a change in diet or a deficit is an empty promise.

Compared with starving oneself for months or years to lose weight, using the potato hack is a whole new kind of dieting experience. The HCG diet uses drops or injections of a human hormone that allow the participant to eat very few calories without feeling hunger. Many people who have tried both the HCG diet and the potato hack have told me that the potato hack has the same effects as the HCG diet, but at a fraction of the cost and without side effects.

> Side effects have also been reported with the HCG diet and include fatigue, irritability, restlessness, depression, fluid buildup (edema), and swelling of the breasts in boys and men (gynecomastia). Another serious concern is the risk of blood clots forming and blocking blood vessels (Mayo Clinic, 2015).

"Fasting" and "cleanses" are an integral part of the dieting landscape lately. These short-term interventions all have great impact, but often are confusing as to what exactly one can eat. The potato hack could be considered a whole-food cleanse, and even a type of monofood fasting.

Weight Loss

The potato hack can be used whether you need to lose 200 pounds or 2 pounds. Many people like to do a round or two of the potato hack in preparation for a class reunion, wedding, or photo-shoot. The fast acting potato hack is absolutely incomparable for losing a few pounds in short order.

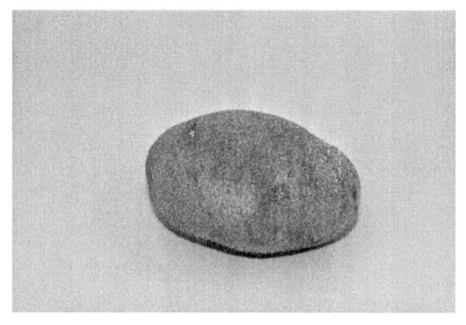

If you have considerably more weight to lose, you will want to do subsequent rounds of the potato hack until your goal weight is reached. Here we'll explore several different ways to pull off these repeated hacks. If your diet is horrendous, i.e. you constantly overeat and traditionally make poor food choices, the potato hack can help get these cravings under control. No amount of potato hacking in the world will overcome bad eating habits, but it may help you see the folly in your ways.

The bane of most diets is that the weight lost comes right back on when you stray from the diet. The potato hack is not a "diet" but a fast fat-reduction method. Fat loss is the end goal of weight loss diets, but the potato hack focuses on this aspect of dieting while keeping your body adequately nourished. If someone were to extract all of the potato's chemicals and put them in a diet pill, it would most likely be the best selling diet pill ever. In food-form, the potato is hands-down the best diet pill ever designed.

Most diets make you focus on a completely new "way of eating," often abbreviated "WOE," and it is indeed woeful to have to learn and adhere to new rules of eating. Diets that make you avoid starches, meat, or fat indefinitely are destined to fail miserably. Our bodies are designed to eat a wide variety of foods. We can only fight nature for so long. Generally, these diets are plagued by strong cravings for forbidden foods, of course if you are reading this, you already know.

Quick Fat Blaster: 1-5 pounds

This is almost *too* easy. As most of you know, losing a pound or two to fit into those skinny jeans can be murder! Not so with the potato hack. You can generally get the results you want in a week. Done just prior to the engagement where you want to look your best, you'll have the added benefit of reduced inflammation giving the appearance of much more weight loss than the scale shows. Many people report much more than weight loss, as well. They stop snoring, have better digestion, and find they are simply not hungry.

The plan: For 3 days, eat nothing but potatoes. Do not fall for the lure of the "variations" I presented earlier. Do this "old school." You have strong *desire* on your side. As legendary waif runway model Kate Moss said:

> Nothing tastes as good as skinny feels (Kate Moss, 2009)

While this statement caused Ms. Moss many years of ridicule, I can see where she was coming from when she said it. Everyone wants to look their best, and when we are forced to parade around in front of old friends, new friends, or judging family, it feels great to be down a few pounds. If you are naturally thin, you won't understand.

Pre-hack – Buy a 20-pound bag of the best potatoes you can find. Organic if possible. Hopefully you know what kind of potatoes you like, having experimented earlier. If you are unsure, I suggest you start with smallish red potatoes. These will be tennis ball sized or smaller. The peels are very thin for easy peeling, if desired. They are very tasty and suited for all recipes.

Day 1 – Pre-cook about 10 pounds of potatoes in any manner you desire following the recipes found here. For breakfast, try the oil-free pan-fried hash browns. For lunch, if you work, pop a couple potatoes in the microwave or just eat them cold. No one will even notice. For dinner, more potatoes, however you like. If you get hungry during the times between meals, keep calm and eat potatoes. Remember, it's not a potato eating contest, it's a fast fat loss diet. Being a bit hungry means you are burning fat. Learn to embrace the hunger and only give in if you must.

Day 2 – Skip breakfast. Maybe gnaw on a small cold potato if you absolutely must, but try waiting as long as possible. Much of the fat loss that occurs on the potato hack happens in that magical time between dinner and your first meal of the day. Extending this time period will lead to more weight loss. Eat a hearty potato lunch. Try a big pile of oven-baked oil-free French fries. Even cold or reheated these taste great. Try not to eat again until dinner. For dinner, eat a hearty serving of potatoes however you like. May I suggest a large serving of mashed potatoes? By now you've tried several recipes, and your pre-cooked potatoes supply is dwindling. On the evening of day 2, cook as many potatoes as you think you'll need for the next day. Go to bed hungry.

Day 3 – Breakfast only if you like. For lunch, a cold boiled potato. Your dinner should be a nice warm potato entrée. Savor the taste. By now you should find yourself actually enjoying a well-prepared potato meal. If you've been choking down cold boiled potatoes, you are undoubtedly getting tired of them. I hope that you try your hand at some of the great recipes provided in this book.

If this is your first try at the potato hack, three days is a great accomplishment! Congratulations. If you are wondering how anybody could eat so many potatoes, remember that in the 1800s potatoes were eaten almost exclusively, even by nobility, in many European countries. The Irish Countess Lady Mountcashel was touring Europe in 1801. A recount of a meeting with a Polish count:

> The more prosperous Irish landowners, on tour in Europe, surprised the continentals by their addiction to potatoes. When the Polish Countess Myscelska called on Lady Mountcashel in Paris, *she found her eating plain boil' d Potatoes for her luncheon in the middle of the day.* She then heard for the first time that that was the principal food of the Irish (Wilmont, C. (1920). *An Irish peer on the Continent (1801-1803)*. Ed. by T. U. Sadlier, London.).

If Lady Mountcashel could do it, so can you! Potatoes are good food.

Day 4 – If you like, add another day to your potato hack, if not, today is your first post-hack day. Eat what you like on this day, but I want you to notice how that first bite of food tastes. Your taste buds and the reward centers of your brain have been numbed by 3 days of bland potatoes. Most likely, you woke up not hungry and, in fact, hungry for potatoes. A great first post-hack meal is hash browns, only this time cooked with a bit of oil and spiced with seasoned-salt. Your taste buds will sparkle as the spices and oil-crisped potatoes slide over your tongue. Have a small piece of chocolate or an orange, you will think you've never had anything so tasty.

Results – If you weighed yourself on Day 1, you should find yourself 2-5 pounds lighter on Day 4. Your clothes will feel looser; people may notice a *leanness* in your face. But best of all, you will have an appreciation for food. A respect for yourself.

> ...but, what is incomparably better, an amount of self-denial which is possessed only by a few (Potato Diet, 1849).

If there's time before your big event, do the potato hack again after a couple days of normal eating. Try one of the variations this time and compare results. Two 3 day hacks a week apart are just perfect for a high school reunion. When people ask how you stay in such good shape, tell 'em, "The potato hack!"

The Stubborn "Last 10"

Whether it's the last 10, 5, or even 2, getting to a goal weight is frustrating. I once spent a full year trying to lose 10 pounds. After two weeks of potato hacking I not only lost those last 10 pounds, but two more. This was back before I tried many other methods and I just powered through, eating plain potatoes day after day as I watched the scale go down, down, down like there was no bottom.

The potato hack will work for you no matter what diet plan got you this far. It may also give you great pause on the wisdom of your current diet. Most diets work great to get you 50-75% of the way to your goal weight, but invariably fall short. As your body weight drops, so does your required caloric intake and also your resting metabolism. You've given your body a lesson in doing more with less and a plateau or stall occurs.

Plateaus are murder for dieters. The normal reaction is to do what you've been doing *harder*. If you've been eating low carb, the tendency is to go lower carb. If you've been eating Weight Watcher, you aim for less points. Hardly ever does this work. The potato hack is a total shock to your system. The anti-inflammatory effects, reward centers, and gut metabolism come into play. Your full belly says "Stop eating!" and your body does not feel starved. Fat burning commences and those final pounds melt away.

The Plan: Start right off with a 5 Day potato hack. Hit your goal weight and stop your crazy dieting! Get your butt into a long-term maintenance plan and forget about your goal weight. Traditional diets that focus on a goal weights, as you'll find, are a fool's game, designed by Big Diet to keep you dieting harder. They know you won't get there. The potato hack is a poke in the eye to Weight Watchers and Jenny Craig. What would Dr. Atkins say if he knew you used evil carbs to beat his carb-phobic diet?

Pre-hack – Buy 30 pounds of the best potatoes you can find. Organic if possible. Try to get a couple different varieties. Search the farmer's markets for heirloom butterfingers, purple Incans, or German reds.

Day 1 – Boil 5 pounds of small potatoes whole following the recipe for "boil'd Potatoes" in the recipe section. After they cool, store them in the fridge. These will be your emergency supply. On Day 1, do it right. No salt, no nuthin'. Just taters. Eat as many times as you want, but remember it's not a potato eatin' contest. Your first day is the toughest, so make a game of it. Cook your potatoes in a variety of ways. Go out and buy a new non-stick pan and some parchment paper if you've found inadequacies in your equipment.

Day 2 – "Second verse, same as the first…little bit louder, little bit worse." Try skipping breakfast. Not mandatory, just an idea. Lots of fat burns while you sleep and it stops when you eat breakfast. Extend the fast and burn more fat. If you find you've already lost a pound or two, high-five yourself. Try eating a couple of the cold boil'd Potatoes during the day, or even for a meal. Day 2 is when you can lose focus. Don't lose focus.

Day 3 – Eat potatoes. OK, you've showed your moxie. Try one of the variations today if you like. If you are digging the weight loss and closing in on that magical goal weight, maybe just keep doin' it 1849 style.

Day 4 – Check your supply of potatoes and pre-cooked "snackers." You don't want to run out today! Get experimental on the recipes. If you are only a pound or two from goal weight, don't do the happy dance just yet. Keep on keepin' on with the spuds. If your friends, family, or coworkers start to take notice of your new potato obsession, tell them all about the potato hack in an Irish accent. Soon you will be the local potato hack guru.

Day 5 – Last day. How'd ya do? If you wake up at goal weight, now is the time for the happy dance. If you still have a ways to go, then maybe just eat up the last of your cold spuds for breakfast and call it quits for this week. Plan on doing it all again next week, you'll have a good idea for how many potatoes you'll need and how many more rounds it will take.

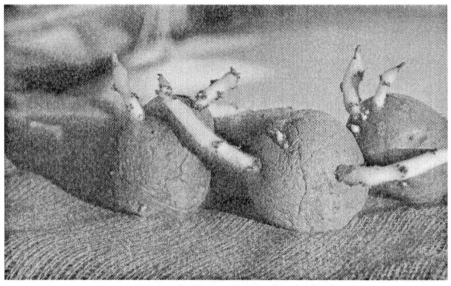

Potatoes Doing the Happy Dance! (Author's Photo)

Results – Most people will lose ½ – 1 pound per day during a 5-day potato hack. Did you meet these expectations? If not, read and re-read the troubleshooting guide at the end. Did you hit your goal weight? If not, will it be worth it to do another round or two? If you hit your weight, make some notes. You will be using the tricks you learned to maintain your weight for the rest of your life.

If you've been dieting for years and stalled for months, you are most likely very happy with me right now. But this was not my doing, it was yours. Pay it forward. Tell all those other unhappy dieters you know about the potato diet, there's enough information in this book that you should be able to talk intelligently about the potato hack. Keep in mind, the last 5 days were how the Irish peasants of 1800 ate every day. If you are planning another week later, are you going to try a variation? Doing it "right" your first week is important, you'll have a baseline for the variations.

First Time Dieters – Twenty to 100+ Pounds

This is for the first time dieters who woke up one day and realized they need to lose some weight. Or possibly the person whose doctor said, "Lose some weight or else!" I love first-time dieters, especially when their heads are not full of stupid advice. The potato hack is all you'll need to make you, and your doctor, very happy. But, my word, you must learn to eat right! If you've been on a diet of Mickey D's for lunch and Taco Bell's "4th meal" for a late night snack, you have a long, long road ahead. The potato diet will help you lose weight and keep it off, but you, my friend, need to learn how to eat.

The Plan: You need a whole new relationship with food, but you don't need to become afraid to eat. Examine your diet. Are you eating enough fruits and vegetables? Are you eating lots of processed foods? Are you a sugar-holic? It's tough to navigate this on your own, so download a couple of diet books. Dr. Phil's 20/20 diet plan is pretty sound, so is the one encouraged by Jack LaLanne in *Live Young Forever*. Stop short of buying into the trademarked diets. If you need to buy special food for the diet to work, it won't work. If you ask me how I eat, I would say that I'm a "vegan who eats meat and a paleo who eats wheat." Getting all religious about a diet plan is the wrong mindset.

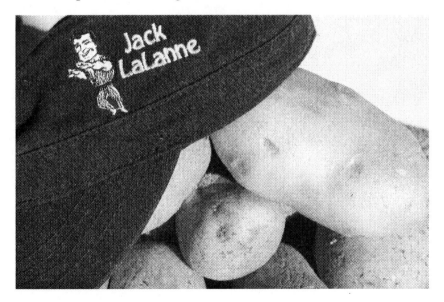

(Author's Photo)

Let's get going on a diet, any diet, and see how you get along. Nearly any diet out there is better than how most Americans eat. The potato hack can help you establish your relationship with food by showing you how delicious real foods are. The potato hack also shows you that "cutting carbs" is a ridiculous idea, especially when wholesome foods such as corn, rice, and potatoes are included in the tally.

> ❝❝ We are far from believing that God created wheat, rye, corn, barley, buckwheat, etc.; chestnuts, beechnuts, butternuts, walnuts, etc., etc.; apples, pears, peaches, plums, grapes, and ten thousand other delicious things, not to be eaten by man (Potato Diet, 1849).

Week 1 – Once you've made up your mind to lose the extra weight, there's no going back. Use this first week to clean house. Get rid of all the junk food and greasy snacks in your house and desk drawers. At some point, buy a 20-pound bag of high-quality, preferably organic, potatoes. Make a couple of the potato dishes from the recipe section and have a couple potato-only meals during the week. Baby steps! Slow and easy wins *this* race.

Week 2 – Try to do a 1-day potato hack. Eat potatoes for breakfast, lunch and dinner. Still hungry? Snack on a potato.

Week 3 through 8 – Try eating "to plan" for the diet you've settled in on. Learn to shop "around the outside" of the grocery store, avoiding the inner aisles filled with processed foods and snacks. Don't bounce back and forth between diet plans, such as low carb and vegetarian. If the plan seems too good to be true, it is. If it seems too difficult, it won't work. This is also the time to evaluate your fitness levels, sleep habits, and stress. A good diet plan will encompass all of these core tenets.

Week 9(ish) – Sometime after you've been eating better for a couple of months, take note of your weight and how you feel. Has two months of the new diet helped you? If you are happy with your new eating style, try a 3-day potato hack to really get things moving. If you are consistently losing 1-3 pounds per week, don't bother with the potato hack. If you've gained weight, re-evaluate everything you are doing.

Weeks 10-26 – After about 6 months of steady dieting, you should be nearing your goal weight. If, along the way, you experience stalls in weight loss that last more than a week or two, throw in a potato hack, as many days as you can stand. This is also a perfect time to try the many variations I showed you. Try some potato-only days or potatoes for breakfast and lunch days. The worst mind-set to get into is one of failure and defeat. If your health seems to be deteriorating, go see a doctor. Maybe you have a health problem.

Weeks 26-52 – As a formerly overweight person, you are hopefully now in "maintenance mode." Be mindful of slipping back into your old habits. Use the potato hack here and there to keep you at your target weight. You may find that your goal weight was too low, and you're better off a bit heavier. Develop life-long eating and fitness habits. Walk every day. Do some strength training.

Results – The potato hack is not a diet, it's a simple hack to help your diet be more effective. As you've read here, the potato hack uses many facets of metabolism and weight loss to help you reset your body and mind to be more receptive to lasting weight loss. Don't be surprised if sometime over the course of the year people start whispering about you, "Is he *sick*?" It's a real shame, but in our society, it seems the only people who lose weight to any degree are the terminally ill. You'll also be asked if you've "had the surgery." Tell them all: "Nope! Just potato hackin.'"

Professional Dieters – Twenty to 100+ Pounds

This is for the folks out there that have spent most of their life dieting. You know all the buzz words. Is your WOE better than SAD? Are you LC or VLC? What did your Ketostix say today? Have you had your BulletProof Coffee® yet? Are you CTing or Grokking the PHD?

Don't worry…I've been there, too. Jumping from diet to diet is a fool's game. Find a good one and stick to it if it makes sense to you. I feel I owe my life to the likes of Mark Sisson, Paul Jaminet, and Dave Asprey… look them up. Let's be clear, there are some exceptional diet plans out there. Almost ALL of them are better than what most Americans eat. The potato hack is not a diet plan. The biggest problem with dieting isn't *losing* weight, it's *keeping it off*. I'm never impressed when someone loses

100 pounds, I'm impressed when they keep 100 pounds off for 5 years. If you've had bariatric or bypass surgery of some type and regained much of the weight, you can use the potato hack to get back down to your desired weight. But you'll need to do a lot of work to learn how to eat right for your body type. There may be underlying medical reasons for your weight gain, i.e. PCOS, thyroid issues, hormonal imbalances, etc... the potato hack will not "fix" any of these, but it may help you to lose weight in spite of your physical impairments and individual genetics.

Bypass surgery poses some unique problems. If you had great success at losing weight immediately after the surgery, much of that success was due to a shift in the gut biome, which is the bacteria in your intestines. Years later, your biome has readapted and could now be holding you back. The potato hack can help to kick-start this process.

Similarly, years spent on trademarked diets like Weight Watchers® or Paleo® may have created a metabolism that is unresponsive to new dietary interventions. You may have developed food allergies from years of avoiding certain foods. Your insulin sensitivity may be poor. You may have developed a condition called, "I-can't-have-that-itis," where you've conditioned yourself to believing that large groups of food are "off-limits." The potato hack just may end up being your best friend.

The Plan: Assess the problem accurately. Get a medical checkup. Ask yourself:

- Am I avoiding any real, whole foods?
- Am I eating processed foods, ie. white flour, sugar, artificial sweeteners, vegetable oils?
- Is my current diet plan working?

If the doctor clears you, maybe it's time for a complete reversal of what you've been doing. Here again is where the potato hack excels. To overcome this syndrome of yo-yo dieting and weight regain, you'll need to adopt a completely different attitude. The potato hack will simply be a tool you carry around in your back pocket to keep you in line. Not a punishment, mind you, but a treat.

> ...all expressed themselves quite satisfied with this diet, and regretted the change back again to the ordinary diet (Potato Hack, 1849).

Week 1 – Jump in with both feet. Do a 3-day potato hack! You're a professional dieter, compare the potato hack to all the other diets you've done. It's undoubtedly healthier than any 3-day intervention you've ever tried. I'm not going to insult your intelligence or berate you, you've had that your whole life, amiright? You may try the potato hack and hate it. No worries. But try it.

Try three full days. Do it 1849-style. Start with 20 pounds of high quality potatoes and work your way through them. Maybe try a variation for a meal or two, but stick to as close a purist approach as possible. You've given other diets their fair due...don't slack on the hack.

Week 2 – Consider last week. How did you do? Did you lose a couple pounds, beat the hunger-monster, or notice anything else? Did you absolutely hate it? If you loved it (or even just kind of liked it) consider what is missing from your normal diet. Are you hungry all the time? Bloated? Do you have poor digestion?

Week 3+ – Consider using the potato hack to augment the diet you are on to see if it benefits you. Consider changing your diet completely and using the potato hack to rest your metabolism. Try all of the variations over the first couple months, see if one suits you better than the others. You are a professional dieter. May the hack be with you!

Results – As much as I hate to say it, some of us will be on a diet for the rest of our lives. I find that using the potato hack to simply augment a pretty good diet works wonders for your attitude and health. The potato hack, as I keep saying, is not a diet, but a tool to use when your normal diet fails you. I'm not naïve, and I know you are not, either. There are many reasons we become overweight and there are major differences in how we respond to diets. Our gender, age, hormonal status, body shape, and genetics all play a role. We'll look next at how to use the potato hack to maintain your weight for life.

Weight Maintenance

The potato hack is second to none for effortlessly maintaining your weight through the years. The goal of every person who has issues with easily gaining weight should be life-long maintenance of their weight in a 5 to 10-pound range. Often when people gain a few pounds over a year or so, it goes unnoticed. After several years, and several pants sizes later, you find that losing those extra 10-20 pounds is not an easy endeavor. The best trick is to not let it get that far out of hand in the first place.

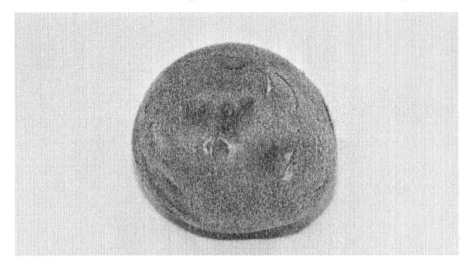

We should all have a subjective measure of our health be it numbers on a scale or the size of our clothes. Scales can be misleading, but if you have a rough idea of what you weigh when you felt healthiest, your weight can be a good indicator of your maintenance activities. Some people do not get along well with scales, they can't handle seeing daily and weekly fluctuations and it causes undue grief. If this is you, throw your scale in the trash and use clothing fit or a "pinch test" to judge your weight.

The plan: Here's where the variations shine. Once you are at or near your goal weight, try a 2 to 3-day potato hack and see how you respond. Try it as they did in 1849 for effect. Once you've done it, plan on using one of the variations periodically for a couple days a month, or even just once a week. Many people will find they can simply eat whatever they like (ehm, within reason) as long as they do a potato hack 2-3 days a month. You won't see big drops on the scale, and may not even notice anything, but you are indeed doing something!

A day of eating only potatoes creates a nice calorie deficit and burns a few ounces of fat. It's always these "few ounces" that sneak up on us. The potato hack is an easy solution. It's not expensive, in fact, cheaper than your normal diet, I'll wager. One of my favorite weight maintenance hacks is "Potatoes by Day (PBD)," found in the variations section. PBD is a hack on another hack called "Vegan Before 6." In VB6, you simply eat nothing but plants during the day and a normal dinner. This is perfectly suited to substituting potatoes for "plants." Just because it's a plant does not mean it will lead to weight loss. For instance, if your VB6 days contain lots of bread, nuts, and fruit it's quite likely your caloric load will be higher. Good vegan diets require a lot of planning and forethought, eating potatoes does not.

Results: The potato hack, with its many variations, should allow you to easily keep your weight in a 5 to 10-pound band year-round, year in and year out. Some like to "hack" before and after the holidays, at the end of summer, end of winter, or whenever you find you've gained a couple pounds. In this regard, no one can say the potato hack is a fad diet. Here we are using the potato hack to simply keep our metabolism, gut health, and weight in check.

Conclusion

For weight loss or maintenance, the potato hack can be a very useful tool. Potato hacking is not a "way of eating," but a way to lose weight and reduce inflammation. The potato hack can augment any weight loss program, or simply be used as a standalone, short-term diet to lose a few pounds, kick-start weight loss, or keep your weight in check year round.

POTATO QUOTES

"NOR DO I SAY IT IS FILTHY TO EAT POTATOES. I DO NOT RIDICULE THE USING OF THEM AS A SAUCE. WHAT I LAUGH AT IS, THE IDEA OF THE USE OF THEM BEING A SAVING. "

WILLIAM COBBETT, BRITISH JOURNALIST (1763?-1835)

Notes:

CHAPTER 4. POTATO HACK RECIPES

You'd think the recipe section for the potato hack would be very small. I'm amazed at how many ways there are to cook dishes in which the only ingredient is potatoes. Many of these will become your "go-to" recipes for *pommes de terre*. This recipe section is divided into four sections: boiled, baked, steamed, and fried. Throughout, the only ingredients I will discuss are potatoes. You can spruce any of these recipes up by using spices of your choosing, if you so desire. I highly, highly recommend that when you first do the potato hack, you try *sans* spices. Salt, OK, a bit. Learning to cook for the potato hack is lots of fun. The recipes are from 200BC up until the late 1800s and today. Per usual, the Irish of old take the grand prize for inventiveness and sheer enjoyment of potatoes.

> There is perhaps no species of food that can be consumed in a greater variety of ways than the potato. Among us the only modes in use are three or four, such as boiling, roasting, or frying (Farmer's Register, Ireland, 1885).

One question I am continually asked is, "Can I eat a raw potato?" The answer is yes. Raw potatoes contain more resistant starch than possibly any food on Earth. A great habit to get into is to eat a slice or two of raw potato any time you are cooking potatoes. This should become a life-long habit, not just a special treat while dieting. Eating a slice raw serves another purpose. If you are unsure of the safety of your potatoes, take a small bite of it raw. If you feel any burning or tingling, this potato could have an unhealthy level of solanine. In the many raw potatoes I've eaten, I've yet to come across one that burns my lips or exhibits signs of high solanine. Raw potatoes are NOT toxic, and in fact, very healthy. However, if all you ate was raw potatoes, you'd get very little nourishment from them as they serve mostly to feed intestinal bacteria, not humans. Besides, they are kind of tasty.

Chuño are potatoes that have been freeze-dried and dehydrated. Originating from the birth-place of the potato high in the Andes Mountains, locals have enjoyed Chuño for thousands of years. Potatoes are laid out on the ground where they freeze at night, the next day they are walked upon to force the juices out and begin drying. The process is repeated for 5 days or more, the result being dried white or black lumps of potato. Chuño could be stored for many years as protection against famine and it was light enough to take on long journeys, only needed to be rehydrated in water. Chuño is available in ethnic stores or on the internet, try some, they make great snacks eaten dry and can be used in many recipes.

For the purpose of this chapter, we'll divide potatoes into five categories:

- Russets (best for baking)
- Whites (best for steaming)
- Reds (best for frying)
- Yellows (best flavor, great for all cooking)
- Blues (all-purpose, fun to eat, hard to find)

Each type is fairly distinguishable, Russets being the typical "baking" potato, oblong with a thick brownish-tan skin. The rest characterized by their color. Within each category is an amazing array of fingerlings, bananas, Finns, butterballs, and new potatoes. In fact, there are over 6000 varieties of potato! Find a good supplier and try them all.

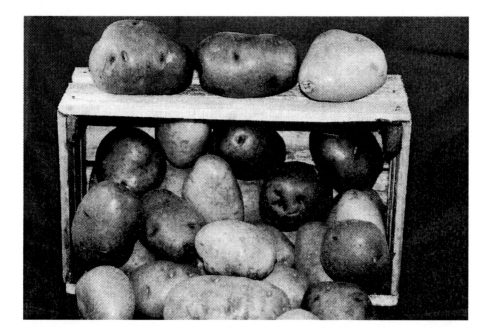

Boiling

Potatoes best suited for boiling are small, thin-skinned potatoes. Reds, yellows, and whites are considered excellent boiling potatoes because they do not disintegrate like the Russets and blues. Choose potatoes that are firm and free of blemishes, eyes, and green spots. Potatoes for boiling should be golf-ball to tennis-ball sized. If bigger, cut into quarters

> Boiling is the simplest, cheapest, and perhaps most nutritious mode of cooking the potato. When boiled, the nourishing substances contained in it are taken into the stomach, more intimately diffused through about three times their weight of water, than is the case with any artificial mixture of the potato-meal and water (Farmer's Register, Ireland, 1885).

Hot Boiled Potatoes

To prepare, simply wash and remove any blemishes, eyes, or green spots. Leave the skin on. If you do not want to eat the peel, it is easily removed after boiling.

- Place your potatoes in a pan of cold water and bring to a boil over medium-high heat.
- Add ½-1tsp of salt to the water if desired while it is boiling.
- Reduce heat to a low boil and cover.
- Boil for 15-20 minutes
- Check for doneness by sticking a potato with a sharp knife, they are done when the knife easily pierces the first 1 inch and meets resistance. Do not overcook!
- When done to the desired consistency, drain the potatoes and eat while hot.

Variation 1: Mashed potatoes. Mashed potatoes are normally made by adding milk and blending or mashing until creamy and smooth. Without milk or butter, you will never get that incredible velvety smoothness you may be used to, but you can mash, even just roughly, into a very decent mashed potato. Required equipment: Potato Masher

Variation 2: Riced potatoes. Potatoes are "riced" by placing them in a special device that forces the potatoes through small holes. The result is a very light and rice-like potato dish. Professional chefs will rice potatoes before mashing to make super-smooth mashed potatoes, but eating freshly riced potatoes is a treat all its own. Required equipment: Potato Ricer

Variation 3: Stone-in-the-Middle. The Irish perfected the cooking of potatoes "with a stone in the middle," meaning they were not cooked completely. This method of cooking maximizes the resistant starch content of the potato. Raw potatoes are extremely high in RS content, but a cooked potato is much more enjoyable to eat.

Proceed as for hot boiled potatoes, but only boil for 10 minutes. The middle should still be uncooked.

Variation 4: Cold "Boil'd" Potatoes. This dish was popularized by the Irish Countess Margaret Mount Cashell in 1800. She enjoyed a lunch of cold Boil'd potatoes [the capital "B" is how they wrote it in

1849!] even when great feasts were presented. By all accounts, she was a beautiful woman. She was noted as "trim and pleasing to the eye," which was quite different from the typical Victorian woman who used a corset to give the appearance of a tiny waist. Perhaps the Countess was potato hacking to maintain her delicate figure.

- Prepare as above, hot or with a stone in the middle.
- When cooked to perfection, drain under cold running water. Cool the potatoes rapidly. When cool to the touch, blot dry and store in the refrigerator.
- Eat with a touch of salt or just plain, as Countess Mount Cashell preferred.

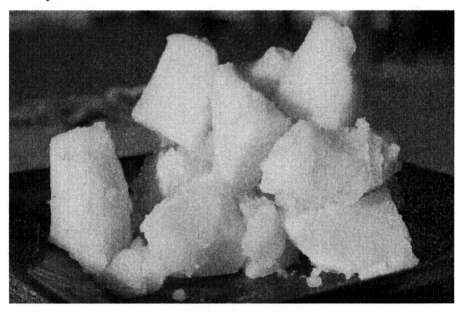

Like Buttah (Photo by Author)

Boil'd potatoes store very well in the refrigerator for up to a week. Much longer and they tend to get rubbery and dry. As with all foods, pay attention to food handling protocols. Do not put hot potatoes into a cold refrigerator; do not leave cooked potatoes at room temperature more than a few hours. To prevent sliced/peeled uncooked potatoes from turning gray keep them in a bowl of cold water until ready for cooking.

Cold boil'd Potatoes make a perfect lunch or midday snack. In fact, cold boil'd Potatoes should make up a large portion of your potato hack days. It's best to pre-cook at least 5-pounds of cold boil'd Potatoes to have on hand for snacking emergencies and quick lunches. If there are other hungry souls about, prepare more, for they will soon be discovered and eaten. Additionally, cold boil'd Potatoes will be used to create several fried and baked dishes later.

Steaming

Steamed potatoes are wonderful to eat plain. This is probably the easiest method of potato preparation as well. If you do not own a steamer, you can make one by placing a metal colander inside of a large pan. Most rice cookers also do a great job of steaming foods.

To steam potatoes, peel if desired—or not. Steam the potatoes for 10-15 minutes, allow to rest a few minutes, and eat. Most recipes call for a 20-minute steam time, I feel this is a bit too long as the shorter time I like leaves the steamed potatoes nice and firm, but please experiment. Allowing the potatoes to cool overnight makes an even better cold potato than when boiled. Steaming keeps much of the potato's crispness intact.

"New" potatoes are small, immature ("baby") potatoes of any variety. They are notoriously hard to cook as they tend to fall apart, especially when boiled. Steaming is by far the best way to cook new potatoes. If you have a hard time eating boiled potatoes, try making a batch of steamed new potatoes. For best results, use potatoes that are ping-pong ball sized, or smaller. New potatoes are perhaps healthier than regular potatoes as they contain all sorts of growth hormones, and steaming helps to preserve their goodness.

Steaming preserves nutrients and minerals perhaps like no other cooking method. Additionally, steamed potatoes can be later fried, roasted, or eaten cold. Steaming is similar to boiling, but anyone who has had both boiled and steamed potatoes will say that steamed are much better.

Baking

Baking refers to cooking potatoes in a hot oven. We could also call this "roasting." Baking imparts a wonderful flavor to plain potatoes. Since man first ate potatoes, they have been baked in one form or another. Historically, potatoes were simply placed next to a fire or put into a pit filled with hot coals and eaten both hot and cold. This method creates many variations of doneness and each potato would taste different, no two alike.

> Throughout all the country it is usual, as every person must have observed, to allow the little children in *every* cottage to *roast potatoes* for their own use, as often as they please, in the turf ashes. As you ride by a cabin, you frequently see a group of children run to the door, each holding in his hand a roasted potato (Farmer's Register, Ireland, 1885).

For baking or roasting, the best potatoes are the stereotypical Russets. Try to get them all in the same size so they cook evenly, and experiment with your oven as temperatures vary greatly. Russets have a nice thick skin that helps impart some flavor in the normally tasteless potato. Russets are not known for their flavor. They fall apart when boiled, but when baked they really shine.

American Style Baked Potato

- Heat oven to 375 degrees. Wrap potatoes in tinfoil and place in hot oven for 60-90 minutes.
- Serve hot

Technically, this produces steamed potatoes, but we call them baked potatoes anyway. It's easy to cook large batches and they store nicely in their little tinfoil wrappings. Eating one is like opening a birthday present. These can be eaten hot or cold, but are probably best when eaten fresh from the oven.

Variation: Cook tin-foil wrapped potatoes in a Crock-pot

English Style Baked Potato (Jacket Potato)

- Poke holes all around the potato with a fork. This will allow the steam to escape, preventing a steamed potato.
- Heat oven to 400 degrees.
- Put the potato straight on the cooking shelf.
- Cook 60-90 minutes and check to see if done by squeezing the potato with an oven-mitted hand. When you sense some "give," it's done.

A properly baked jacket potato will have a crispy crunchy skin and fluffy insides. Americans usually eat baked potatoes with sour cream, butter, and maybe some bacon. The Brits are a bit more inventive, serving their perfectly baked jacket potatoes as a main meal filled with wonderful things like prawns, fish, cheese, eggs, chutney, or simply butter, salt and pepper. For the potato hack, we'll go light on the toppings and just eat them straight from the oven. Put the uneaten baked potatoes in the fridge for another day.

Variation 1: Cook jacket potatoes in the microwave. Not quite as crunchy, but OK in a pinch. Be sure to poke with a fork before cooking or you'll have a mess on your hands.

Variation 2: Cut the potato into quarters and bake in the same way. The result is oven-baked "French fries" to die for. This is the traditional "jojo" potato, invented in Elyria, Ohio.

Variation 3: Cook in a wood fire. If you heat with a wood stove, or build the occasional bon fire, toss in a bunch of potatoes and eat them really "old school." You'll be amazed at the flavors picked up from the ashes and dirt.

Irish Roasted Potatoes

These you will want to make over and over. Leave it to the Irish to out-do the English in potato cuisine, right? Choose a bit smaller potatoes. Russets are still the best choice. Get Prince Edward Island (PEI) Russets specifically for a treat you will not soon forget.

- Preheat oven to 425 degrees.

- Peel your potatoes and drop into boiling water for exactly 7 minutes. You'll know their ready when the outer ¼ – ½ inch is cooked, but the rest is still raw. This is known as parboiling.

- Drain the potatoes in a strainer or by using the lid to hold the potatoes while dumping the water.

- Now here's the important part, you gotta "rough 'em up." Leave it to the fightin' Irish to force their potatoes into tasting good, but this roughing-up is crucial. Give the cooked potatoes a thorough shaking in the empty pan, don't be gentle. They should look like they were trampled on by a stampede of drunk Irish partiers.

- Once thoroughly roughed-up, place the potatoes on cookie tray or baking dish lined with parchment paper. The traditional way (remember this for later!) is to fry them quickly in a bit of duck fat or grease first, and then roast. Using parchment paper in a very hot oven will brown them nicely without using oil.

- Half-way through their cooking, turn the potatoes to brown them evenly.

- Cook about 60 minutes until browned.

- Eat hot, save the leftovers. Potatoes roasted in this manner are traditionally eaten as-is, or with a bit of gravy…the perfect accompaniment to roast beef or turkey.

Variation 1: Use leftover boiled potatoes in place of parboiled potatoes. They turn out surprisingly well especially if cooked on parchment paper in a very hot oven. Don't overcook, and don't be afraid to *rough them up a bit.*

Variation 2: Cut fresh, parboiled, or leftover boiled potatoes into cubes or strips. Bake at the same high heat on parchment paper, turning midway through. Thank me later.

Frying

By now you must think me totally mad, but I'm going to give you several oil-less methods of frying potatoes that will make your mouth water. First, some mandatory equipment. You'll need a really good non-stick pan. I do not recommend Teflon, but if you are comfortable, go ahead. I prefer ceramic non-stick or any of the newer non-Teflon types. Look for a pan that says "PTFE-Free, PFOA-Free, and Cadmium-Free." Even a properly seasoned cast-iron or stainless steel pan will work, maybe even better. The key is a good non-stick pan and lower heat than you are used to.

The best potatoes for frying are the reds. They can take a good bit of heat without scorching and they brown up nicely in a frying pan. Back in my Fry Daddy phase, I was amazed one day when I mixed together freshly cut red and white potatoes. After a couple minutes in the fryer, the white potatoes were nearly burnt while the reds were still a bright white.

Hash Browns

Hash browns are potatoes that have been shredded, julienned, diced, or riced and fried, usually in really bad oil. These are the mainstay of the "greasy spoon" diners and truck stops across America. I used to love hash browns at popular breakfast spots like Denny's and IHOPs, but now they just taste like a sponge soaked in Wesson oil. Admittedly, the best hash browns are fried in bacon grease, butter, or coconut oil, and some people have tweaked the potato hack to include these, but with the proper pan, oil is not needed. Oil-less hash browns will give you a whole new perspective on how tasty potatoes can be.

First shred some raw potatoes. Use a cheap box-type shredder, a fancy one made just for potatoes, or a food processor. Try shredding the potatoes into different sizes, each way of shredding cooks a bit differently and you may develop a preference. I like thickly shredded potatoes.

Pre-heat your pan over medium heat. The pan not be too hot or they will scorch and ruin the meal. Put your potatoes in and cover for about 10 minutes. You may hear some sizzling, but you should not smell burned potatoes. Flip and repeat. After turning, you can increase the heat slightly. Keep covered. After 5 or 6 minutes, check them with your spatula.

You should be able to flip them like a pancake, but if there are too many, you can just flip in a haphazard fashion.

Hash browns are done when both sides are browned nicely and the center is still gooey. Slide onto a plate and *bon appétit*. If I weren't such a stickler for the potato hack, I'd sneak on some salt, pepper and vinegar (you did not hear that from me!).

Variation 1: Baked Hash Browns. Place a pile of shredded hash browns on a parchment paper lined cookie tray and bake at 400-450 for 20-30 minutes.

Variation 2: Curly fries! These great novelty fries will make you think of county fairs and circuses. You'll need a curly fry cutter, sold on Amazon as "Tater Twisters" or "Spiral Slicers." Simply cut up a potato using whatever system you find useful and pile in a frying pan and cook just like hash browns.

Home Fries

I remember my first trip away from Ohio. The waitress asked, "Hash browns or home fries?" I knew what hash browns were, heck, I even knew what jojo potatoes were, but never heard of home fries. Home fries, as it turns out, are cubed potatoes cooked like hash browns. This is now one of my favorite ways to cook potatoes. Cubing can be done with a knife, but it's time consuming to get them small enough. Home fries come frozen in bags, which may be the easiest way. I prefer to cut them by hand.

Once you cubed a couple of raw potatoes (or cheat and use frozen), cook them like hashbrowns. If they are very fresh potatoes, the cubes will stick together as the starch coagulates and you can flip them in one piece. The frozen varieties always tend to cook individually and you more "stir-fry" than flip. Either way, they cook up perfectly in an un-oiled non-stick pan. Cook to desired doneness.

Variation 1: Baked Home Fries. Cook in a 400 to 450-degree oven on parchment paper for 20-30 minutes.

Variation 2: Instead of fresh potatoes, use your cold Boil'd potatoes. Cook them in your non-stick pan just like hash browns and home fries. Stir frequently and since they are already cooked; just heat until browned.

Potato Baklava

You could also call this "potato chip pie." Baklava is a Turkish dessert made by layering dozens of sheets of paper-thin pastry (filo) dough upon one another and interspersed with nuts and honey, basically. It's the many layers that make it so unique, like the thousands of folds and layers in a Samurai sword, I suppose. Anyhoo, you can do it with potatoes, too (sans honey and nuts, of course).

- You'll need an inexpensive mandolin, and some Band-Aids if you have not used a mandolin before. I wear a heavy oven mitt when using mine. You'll see.
- Slice raw potatoes with your mandolin and place in your pre-heated, medium hot frying pan. Move around as you slice to form layer-upon-layer of paper thin potato slices. You'll want 10-15 layers.
- Cover and let the bottom brown a bit, then flip and cook the other side. Turn up heat just a tad and flip again.
- Keep flipping until you get the desired brownness.

Regular fried potatoes, the kind that are about ¼" thick, do not lend themselves well to no-oil frying, but you may have success. The thinness of baklava potatoes makes them an absolute treat to eat, even when cold the next day.

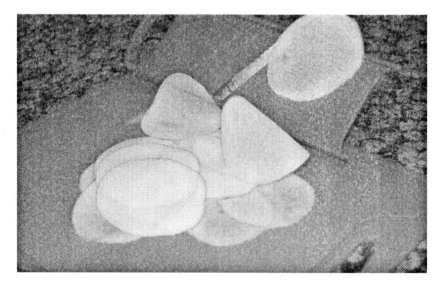

Mandolin Slicer (Author's Photo)

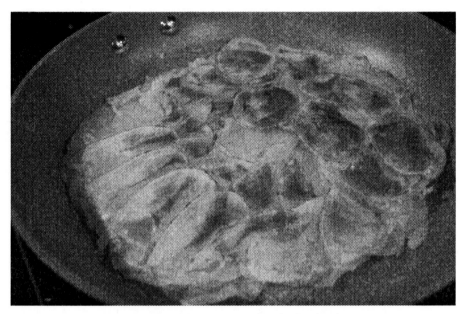

No-oil Baklava Potatoes (Author's Photo)

For the "cheaters"

I've given you all many, many ways to cook potatoes for the potato hack. Try them all. Once you start braving out on your own and playing with the variations to the potato hack, you'll find you can make really tasty potato dishes for the whole family with no oil. Mashed potatoes can be made super-palatable with a cup of chicken broth, and a nice gravy can be made with chicken broth and potato starch. I will give in and admit that many of these potato dishes are a bit on the dry side and some gravy can liven up meals enough that you can stick with the hack indefinitely. Most assuredly, shortly after man discovered potatoes, he invented gravy.

Potato Starch Gravy Recipe

Ingredients:

- 2 cups chicken broth
- 1TBS potato starch
- Salt&pepper to taste

Directions:

Heat 1½ cup of the broth to boiling. While waiting for the broth to boil, mix the potato starch with ½ cup of cold broth. Whisk well. As soon as the broth has come to a full boil, remove from heat and quickly stir in the well-mixed potato starch. The potato starch will instantly gel and form a nice, thick gravy. Season as desired.

> For it must be a considerable time before the English people can be brought to eat potatoes in the Irish style; that is to say, scratch them out of the earth with their paws, toss them into a pot without washing, and when boiled, turn them out on a dirty board, and then sit round that board, peel the skin and dirt from one at a time, and eat the inside! (Farmer's Register, Ireland, 1885).

POTATO QUOTES

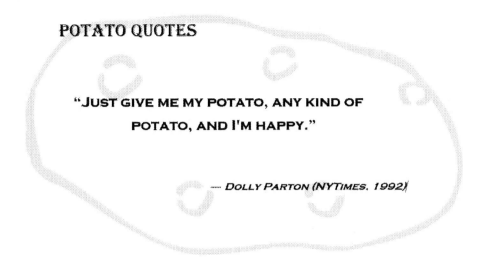

"JUST GIVE ME MY POTATO, ANY KIND OF POTATO, AND I'M HAPPY."

—— DOLLY PARTON (NYTIMES. 1992)

Notes:

CHAPTER 5. TROUBLESHOOTING

If I told you that the potato hack works perfectly for everyone I'd be just as big a liar as those folks with the trademarked diets. No diet works perfectly for everyone, just as no medicine works perfectly for everyone. If diet gurus had to follow the same rules as Big Pharma, the lists of side-effects would scare everyone off of dieting forever. Low carb diets can cause brain fog, nausea, diarrhea, or constipation. High protein diets can cause kidney problems, bad breath, and even cancer. No diet is without risk, but perhaps the worst "diet" is the one that nearly everyone in the "civilized" world is on, the Western Diet. The potato hack is not without side-effects for some, and it sometimes falls short of the promise of rapid weight loss and improved digestion. In this chapter, we'll take a look at some of the common problems as we troubleshoot a solution.

Side-effects

- Hyperglycemia
- Hypoglycemia
- Nausea
- Itching and Swelling
- Windiness
- Weight gain
- Lack of weight loss
- Hunger

The most common side effects are hunger and failure to lose weight. The side-effects of the potato hack can be deadly in some circumstances, so let's explore, starting with the most dangerous.

Hyperglycemia

Hyperglycemia (high blood sugar) is a condition in which blood sugar levels rise too high following a meal containing carbohydrates. Most likely, if you are diabetic or even pre-diabetic, you knew about it long before you picked up a copy of The Potato Hack, but many people walk around unaware they have a problem with blood sugar.

If you experience any of the following after an all-potato meal, please get to a doctor and have your blood glucose tested, it could save your life.

- blurry vision
- difficulty concentrating
- frequent urination
- headaches
- increased fatigue
- increased thirst

These are all symptoms of hyperglycemia, a condition in which your blood glucose stays above 200 milligrams per deciliter (mg/dL), or 11 millimoles per liter (mmol/L). Normal ranges of blood glucose following a starchy meal are in the 110 to 180 mg/dL range as measured with a simple home blood glucose monitor. If you are concerned that you have blood glucose issues, the potato hack can be used as a test.

There are two types of diabetes. Type 1 Diabetes (T1D) occurs when your pancreas fails to produce insulin, this condition necessitates the use of insulin shots to maintain blood sugar levels. If you have T1D, chances are you are not just now finding out. The other type of diabetes is Type 2 Diabetes (T2D) in which either your pancreas produces too little or your body in no longer sensitive to insulin. Pre-diabetes is the condition where you are having insulin sensitivity, but your levels do not yet call for insulin injections or medications.

Again, I stress, if you think you are having blood glucose issues, GO TO THE DOCTOR. But if you are just curious as to what kind of glucose control you have, here's what you can do. Purchase a cheap home glucose test kit, the type diabetics use. They can be purchased without a prescription at any drug store or on Amazon. If the kit does not come with test strips, you'll need to buy some. The test strips usually come in packets of 25-50. Get 50. Learn to use your new toy. Read the directions.

Most meters need to be calibrated first, the instructions will explain how. Once you are comfortable poking yourself with the tiny needle and reading the meter, it's time to proceed.

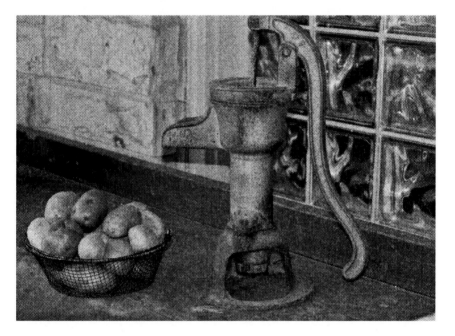

Doctors use what is called an oral glucose tolerance test (OGTT). They give you a super-sweet drink that has a certain dose of a sugar called glucose. When you drink it, your body should sense the sugar rush and prompt your pancreas to produce insulin. The infusion of insulin causes cells in your body to "open up" and absorb the glucose in your blood. When you do not produce adequate insulin, or your cells are "insulin resistant," the glucose stays in your blood. A buildup of glucose in your blood is toxic to many organs, including your brain.

As far as the potato hack goes, the big concern is those that are pre-diabetic, or even full-blown T2D, but don't know it. Many, if not most, obese people are insulin resistant and possibly pre-diabetic. To perform your own OGTT, simply test your blood glucose with your new meter throughout the day, but be methodical otherwise the numbers are meaningless. First, though, get a baseline for what your fasting blood glucose (FBG) is. FBG is your glucose level when you first wake up in the morning. Take a reading several mornings in a row and record them on a sheet of paper, or in a spreadsheet on your computer. Normal readings will be in the 70-100 range, preferably below 90. Also, periodically through the week, test your blood glucose at one and two-hours after a meal. Normal ranges will be 110 to 200, preferably below 140. If you have FBGs every morning of 130 or higher, or if your postprandial (after-meal) readings are above 200, do not proceed, go to the doctor for advice and then read everything you can on the subject. If your FBG is in the normal range, proceed with the potato hack OGTT.

On the morning of your test, record your FBG. Take a new reading every 30 minutes until you eat your first meal and write them down. At your first meal, eat about 1 pound of plain potato, especially be sure to not put any vinegar on the potato as this can affect postprandial glucose. After your meal, take a blood glucose reading every 15 minutes for three hours. Then every 30 minutes for another two hours if things have leveled out. What you will see is a chart like this:

Time	Blood Glucose
7:00 (FBG)	85
7:30	80
8:00	76
8:30 (eat potato)	100
8:45	120
9:00	125
9:15	140
9:30	135
9:45	135
10:00	120
10:15	105
10:30	90
10:45	83
11:00	70
11:15	75
11:30	70
12:00	70
12:30	66
13:00 (stop test)	64

Upon examination, you can see why taking the readings at exactly one – and two-hours could be misleading. In this example of a perfectly normal glucose curve, we see that the highest peak was at 9:15, 45 minutes after the meal. Then a steady decline as the glucose from the potato entered cells in your muscles and organs. The low readings just before lunch are normal, sometimes referred to as a "sugar crash." This explains the drowsiness and lethargy sometimes felt when you know you need to eat something. The normal, healthy body keeps amazingly tight control of blood glucose, but things can go awry, as in this table:

Time	Blood Glucose
7:00 (FBG)	128
7:30	120
8:00	120
8:30 (eat potato)	120
8:45	140
9:00	155
9:15	180
9:30	220
9:45	267
10:00	300
10:15	345
10:30	415
10:45	415
11:00	400
11:15	400
11:30	376
12:00	350
12:30	350
13:00 (stop test)	325

If your numbers look like this, well, sorry. You have Type 2 Diabetes. Your FBG in this case indicates almost "pre-diabetic" but the potato hack OGTT indicates full-fledged T2D. Go to the doctor! Show him the results, and learn to deal with your newly diagnosed disease. This is not something you want to play with. Type 2 Diabetes can sometimes be controlled with diet, but may require medication.

The population I am concerned mostly with regarding blood sugar control are those who have been following a low-carb or ketogenic diet for a long time. The diet may be covering up hidden blood glucose issues or may be inducing a condition known as "physiological insulin resistance" caused when you do not ingest dietary carbs and your body loses the ability to control them when eaten. This physiological insulin resistance is a common occurrence in low-carb circles, so it may be wise to play around a bit eating higher carbs than normal to reverse it. Your glucose testing meter and strips will help you to determine the severity of your insulin resistance in any case.

Hypoglycemia

Hypoglycemia (low blood sugar) is the exact opposite of the hyperglycemia seen in diabetes. Generally, hypoglycemia is seen in people being treated for diabetes, but it can also occur in normal, healthy people following a very carb-heavy meal. Symptoms associated with hypoglycemia are:

- Heart palpitations
- Fatigue
- Pale skin
- Shakiness
- Anxiety
- Sweating
- Hunger
- Irritability
- Tingling sensation around the mouth
- Crying out during sleep

If you experience these on the potato hack, you should go to the doctor immediately. Chances are, however, that if you have this condition, you already know. What can happen, however, on the potato hack, is that people are simply used to eating so often and never experience a normal drop in blood sugar as we noticed on the blood-glucose charts. This is known as reactive or postprandial hypoglycemia and quite possibly shocking the first time you feel it. Generally, reactive hypoglycemia simply results in a feeling of light-headedness or dizziness. If you were to check your blood glucose level with a test meter, you'd see a reading of 50-60 mg/dL. This can be quickly rectified by eating a potato.

The potato hack is a hack on insulin sensitivity. For people with low insulin sensitivity, drastic improvements can be had in as little as one day. In the days before test meters and Metformin, doctors used a potato diet to treat diabetes with great success. Many people who have tried the potato hack report that their FBGs have gone from pre-diabetic to normal in just one day and that postprandial readings drop considerably even after they are done with the hack. Insulin sensitivity is the holy grail of metabolic health. The potato hack can help to improve insulin sensitivity in the majority of people, however for those with seriously impaired glucose control issues, the potato hack may uncover something sinister.

Nausea

Occasionally someone will report that they've eaten a meal of potatoes and suddenly felt nauseous. Sometimes this happens after an extremely large meal, much bigger that the meals they are used to eating, but sometimes just out-of-the-blue. Early in my dieting "career," I read that coconut oil is extremely healthy and can lead to quick weight loss. The recommendation was to eat several spoonful's a day. The first time I tried, I became instantly nauseated and nearly puked. A quick visit to "Dr. Google" and I found that nausea is a common side effect of coconut oil consumption, with no good explanation for why.

I have a theory. People with compromised guts, i.e. IBS, SIBO, or "leaky gut" are very sensitive to certain foods. While it's rare to hear anyone ever say that potatoes make them feel nauseous, it's not uncommon to hear this in dieting circles. If potatoes were commonly nauseating, McDonald's would not be selling billions of orders of fries every day. When the lining of a person's gut is compromised, ingestion of certain food causes the feeling of nausea, often followed by diarrhea or vomiting just as if they had consumed rotten food.

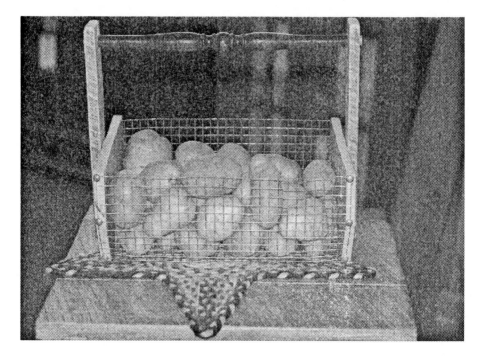

Our body has a very good system in place to expel any food that can do it harm. The colon can flood itself with water in an instant to create explosive diarrhea. People with compromised guts are sensitive to many more foods than other people. Normally healthy foods, like coconut oil, can make someone with an injured gut very queasy. Potatoes contain a compound called "lectins." Normally these lectins are reduced by stomach acid and digestive enzymes. If someone has a less than stellar digestive system, as comes from years of food avoidance or a medical condition, then the lectins may not be destroyed before entering the colon, and nausea ensues.

If you have a sensitive digestive system, get frequent heartburn, nausea, indigestion, upset, stomach, or diarrhea, aka "The Modern Dyspeptic Gut," then don't be surprised if the potato hack gives you some of the same complaints. The irony in this is, the cure may be found in the potato hack itself. It may be your normal diet that is causing the problems. Many times people end up eating only the things they can tolerate and this leads to more and more food sensitivities. Better is to diversify the diet until more and more foods can be eaten with no ill effect. The potato hack is a gut-strengthening elimination diet. Perhaps those with the modern dyspeptic gut should consider potato hacking intermittently until their guts are stronger.

On the other hand, nausea after a potato-only meal could mean something entirely different. Potatoes are food. Food can "go bad." Cooked potatoes left overnight at room temperature could easily grow mold or attract harmful bacteria. When eaten, these potatoes could cause food poisoning. Mild cases of food poisoning are usually described as nausea. In worse cases, diarrhea and vomiting. Most cases of food poisoning resolve on their own without medical interventions. If your nausea turns to vomiting and diarrhea and you are becoming weak and dehydrated, it would be wise to seek medical attention.

In essence then, nausea could be caused by two things:

- A normal potato and an abnormal gut
- An abnormal potato and a normal gut

Itching and Swelling

Itching and swelling are classic signs of a food allergy. As potatoes are so common in our daily lives, it would surprise me to hear of someone learning of a potato allergy when trying the potato hack. However, it would not surprise me to hear that someone who had rarely handled raw potatoes had a reaction.

The most troubling compounds (i.e. solanine) are found mostly in the skin and sprouts of a potato. Store-bought potatoes are regulated as to how much solanine they may contain. Handling, that is, washing, peeling, and cutting, rarely produce allergic reactions. Heirloom varieties like you may grow yourself or buy at a farmer's market could possibly contain lethal amounts of solanine. While it would be rare, unheard of, really, it's possible that a potato could develop high levels of solanine. When peeling such a potato, it would cause an allergic reaction such as itching and redness if the juice were to get on your skin.

If you experience itching and swelling while handling a potato, best to toss that one (or the whole batch) in the trash. If you experience body-wide itching, hives, or swelling after eating potatoes, you may wish to visit an allergy specialist to rule out a potato allergy.

Windiness

OK, let's just come out and say it. Fart. Potatoes might make you fart. If lots of foods tend to make you fart, the potato hack undoubtedly will, too. Farts were probably not vilified nor a cause of ridicule until our diet changed drastically in the past couple hundred years. Any population eating a diet with lots of fermentable fiber be it from meat or plant, would be a population that knows gas. A diet that produces little gas, or intermittent levels of gas with asphyxiating properties, is not a diet that favors good populations of gut microbes. No one cringes and points fingers when a person sneezes, so should it be with the common fart.

If you find yourself farting continuously after a meal of potatoes, it's not the potato's fault. It's your fault. Your diet is most assuredly lacking in fiber, specifically, fermentable, prebiotic fiber. Potatoes are an exceptional source of fiber. To be ashamed of their wind-generation capabilities is a disservice to the potato and your intestines.

If you cannot take the farts, try instead a slower approach. Try one of the variations such as PUDDD or PBD. Work your way up to a full day of potatoes. This is another perfect example of a potato hack side effect being treated with the potato hack itself.

Weight gain

Throughout the book, I use the terms "weight gain" and "weight loss" to be synonymous with "fat gain and fat loss." What we are after with the potato hack, mainly, is *fat* loss. It's hard to measure actual fat loss, so we use weight as a proxy for measuring fat. This is often misleading. You can lose fat while gaining weight, or gain fat while losing weight. Let me explain.

By most accounts our body is 60% water by weight. A 140-pound person has roughly 84 pounds of water in their body. Through food and drink, we ingest an additional 3 to 5-pounds of water every day. Most of this water is eliminated in urine and sweat, but some of it can stick around. Ladies all know what happens during their monthly cycles; they gain weight. Pre-menstrual weight gains of 3-7 pounds are the norm. This is simple water retention due to shifting hormone levels. Any human at any time can have similar fluctuations that result in water retention.

What I am describing here is different from "chronic water retention" which is usually the result of poor kidney function or chronic hormonal imbalances. Potato hackers often come screaming through my door on day two saying that they've gained 2, 3, or 4 pounds *overnight*. This is one of those WTF (where's the fudge?) moments for potato hackers hoping to wake up 5-pounds lighter. Have no fear, though. This overnight weight gain is not fat…it can't be. If you only ate 1400 or less calories the day prior, and gained weight, it's water.

Most of the complainants of weight gain are ladies. If ladies are not used to weighing daily, they are often surprised by how much their weight actually fluctuates in the week or so preceding a period. Guys, on the other hand, can fluctuate from eating too much salt, exercising too much, or simply from being *around* a woman about to go on her period (OK, I made that one up).

The potato hack is anti-inflammatory by nature. Potatoes contain several anti-inflammatory compounds that tend to reduce any hidden, chronic inflammation a person has. Once this inflammation is reduced, the potato hack really works well. Some folks might have an inflammatory disease such as arthritis or hay fever. The potato hack usually works wonders for reducing this type of inflammation, but there is always room for a condition that the potato hack cannot overcome.

My recommendations for anyone who gains weight with the potato hack:

- Stop at first sign of weight gain and return to your normal diet, or
- Ignore the weight gain and press on with the potato hack, or
- Ignore the weight gain for two days and reevaluate

There is no shame in calling the potato hack a failure for you. As I've said before, there is no one-size-fits-all diet. Lots of times the weight loss with the potato hack is not linear. Which brings us to the next side effect.

Lack of Weight Loss

Just as frustrating as weight gain is failure to lose. You've been promised an amazing ½ to 1-pound weight loss per day, yet on day 3 you are at your same starting weight. WTF (where's the fudge)?

I've talked with hundreds of people doing short-term and long-term potato hacks. I will say without hesitation that the lasting results are in the ½ to 1-pound per day range, but the weight lost is not always linear. People love to post their daily stats when potato hacking, just Google "potato hack results" and you'll see what I mean. Most often, the results look like this:

Starting weight 208.

- Day 1 – 208
- Day 2 – 209
- Day 3 – 206
- Day 4 – 205
- Day 5 – 205

This represents an overall weight loss of 3 pounds over 5 days. But what it even more represents is someone who is doing the potato hack and losing fat at an undisclosed rate. If 208 is an actual valid starting weight and 205 an actual valid ending weight, 3-pounds over 5-days is a decent weight loss, and most likely is truly all weight from body fat. However, the starting weight may be a bit skewed depending on time of day, time of month, or even the previous day's food intake. Many, many people have reported back a week after their potato hack experiment to brag about an additional 2-3 pounds lost in the following week while eating their regular diet. In fact, this is such a common occurrence it's expected.

For someone following the "Fat Blasting" protocol of potato hacking, they will be ecstatic with 3-pounds in 5-days and will most likely do another round later. For someone with 100 pounds to lose, it may seem like a dismal return for eating *potatoes*. Judging from the headlines of popular fitness magazines, a diet should promise "10 pounds in 10 days," or "20 pounds a month!" to be any good. These diets are all hype. A pound a day for 10 days is water that you'll gain right back.

The best method of losing weight is *slowly*. Three to five pounds per week is the recommended safe zone for weight loss. The potato hack is perfect for this type of weight loss. For those with 10+ pounds to lose, simply track your weight randomly throughout the week. Eventually you will see patterns and your daily lows will become your daily highs and soon you will be seeing numbers you have not seen for a long time. I remember when I was dieting, I had not seen 190 in close to 10 years, 180 in 15 years, and 170 in nearly two decades. The potato diet allowed me to not only hit my goal weight of 170, but knock off an additional

10-pounds to see my lowest adult weight in over 25 years.

On the other hand, if you look at the 1840's Prison Diet Experiments, you'll note that most of the prisoners gained weight on 6 pounds of potatoes per day. Most likely these poor souls were all starving and malnourished, the potato meals being quite better than what they were eating beforehand. But the fact is, they gained weight eating potatoes. You can, too! It's not likely anyone will gain much weight eating 3-5 pounds of potatoes a day, but it's possible. If you are a small person who normally eats only 1200 calories per day and you start eating 1500 calories of potatoes, you just might be in for a surprise.

The potato hack will test your will to lose weight for sure. You may find that you are so addicted to the processed treats we're all confronted with to give them up. If you are not losing weight with the potato hack, ask yourself:

- Have you given it enough time?
- Are you really doing the potato diet, or a variation of your own?
- Are you simply enjoying potatoes too much and overeating?

The failure to lose weight may be a reason for you to never try the potato hack again. No shame in that, as long as you gave it a good try. There's always Weight Watchers®.

Hunger

The potato hack promises HCG-like levels of non-hunger, but just Google "HCG diet and hunger" and you will see a recurrent theme… HCG dieters are hungry, too. Notice that hunger is last in my list of side effects. Hunger is good. Hunger means your body is alive. The average Westerner in 2016 just does not know what hunger is. Use your time with the potato hack to understand hunger.

Make it a game. A "hunger game" if you will. Tell yourself, "I will eat nothing but nourishing potatoes for X days." Then see how long you can last. Most people have no problem lasting 3-5 days. One to two days is child's play. Seven to fourteen days is tough. I can personally vouch, having done 14 days.

Confucius taught a practice known as *Hara Hachi Bu*. The goal being to eat until 80% full. *Hara Hachi Bu* has been studied by many scientists and is believed to possess many properties that keep people thin. Calorie restriction, hunger hormones, stomach stretching signals and other core tenets of the potato hack all come into play with *Hara Hachi Bu*.

My recommendations for folks who are constantly hungry while potato hacking:

- *Hara Hachi Bu*
- Hunger games
- Stop the potato hack

Use the potato hack to get to know hunger, you may like him. Hunger is one of those strange automatic signals our body produces that we have complete control over. Your body says, "I'm hungry." But you don't have to feed it.

Conclusion

Not everyone who tries the potato hack is going to succeed. If you gave it a good try and failed, don't feel bad. Maybe your body is trying to tell you something. Do you need more fiber in your diet? Have you adopted horrible eating practices over the years? While eating should not be so hard, these days it can be impossible to understand what is hype and what is good advice. If you want a diet overhaul, first give up processed foods that contain sugar, oil, and wheat. Do not replace these foods with healthier gluten-free, low-fat, sugar free alternatives, but replace them with real food, ie. apples, bananas, and honey. Many of my friends are calling this the "SOW" diet (sugar, oil, wheat).

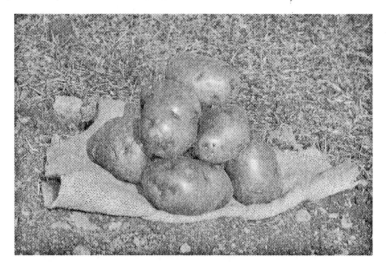

POTATO QUOTES

"THE POTATO IS CRITICISED WITH REASON FOR BEING WINDY, BUT WHAT MATTERS WINDINESS FOR THE VIGOROUS ORGANISIMS OF PEASANTS AND LABOURERS?"

DENIS DIDEROT (1713-1784),' L'ENCYCLOPEDIE' (1751-1772)

Notes:

PART 2

ALL ABOUT POTATOES

Chapter 6. Potatoes: The Good, the Bad, and the Ugly

Invariably when I start to talk about the potato hack, a hand goes up. "Can I use bananas instead of potatoes?" "What about using broccoli or beans?"

Generally, I try to give a polite answer, pointing out that there is no historical precedence for such a diet, but that it *just might* work. Of course, it would no longer be the *potato* hack, but some other hack. I then recommend they search for historical references and spend a couple years experimenting. I have no doubt that there are foods that will exert a similar effect, but I've not found them. I once tried a week-long "bean hack" and it did not go so well.

I have empathy for people who *can't* eat potatoes. This is different than people who *don't* eat potatoes. Potatoes are a member of the nightshade family of plants, and some people are allergic to potatoes (as well as peppers, tomatoes, and eggplant). I rarely hear from people with nightshade allergies as the potato hack is about as appealing to them as "free peanuts for life" are to someone with peanut allergies.

Then there are people who *don't* eat potatoes. They've been convinced that potatoes are simple "carbs" that lead to weight gain and metabolic syndrome. Loren Cordain, the Paleo Diet® guru, says of potatoes, "… in effect, eating potatoes is a lot like eating pure sugars, but even worse, in terms of the harm these starchy tubers do to our blood sugar levels." Many millions of people have heard this and similar warnings that potatoes are somehow bad for us. I myself stopped eating potatoes for nearly two years because I drank the Koolaid that said "carbs are evil."

Low carb diets have become all the rage, and the poster child for a "carb" is, unfortunately, the potato. Well, low-carbers of the world… here's a challenge. Try the potato hack for 3 days. It may just change your life! When I tried a low carb diet, the very first foods to go were beans, rice, and potatoes. These foods are easily identified as "carbs," and it seems such a good idea to avoid them all. But in a "whole food" sense, beans, rice, and potatoes have it all. Trust me…beans, rice, and potatoes are not the enemy.

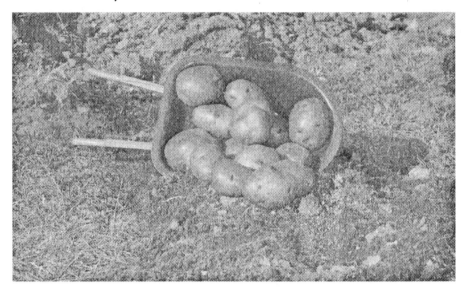

Why Potatoes?

Believe it or not, I didn't just pick potatoes out of thin air. It was a long journey. I first read about a man named Chris Voigt, Commissioner of the Washington State Potato Board, who was doing a publicity campaign for potatoes. Dr. Voight ate potatoes for 60 days straight. All of the news outlets picked up on his story and many articles were written about his experience (More on Voigt in the "Icons" chapter). Later, a friend forwarded me the 1849 *Water-cure Journal* article "Potato Diet." With these in mind, I Googled "Potato Diet" and only found a few crazed bloggers discussing a possible potato diet. Other than the few obscure references discussed, I was on my own in vetting the potato hack. The Interwebz were of little help.

When I started searching scholarly research journals, I found a plethora of studies that dissected the unique nutrition qualities of the potato. For three years, I studied potatoes and their "magic." I formulated the potato hack based on the experiences of hundreds of people that I convinced to try a potato-only diet. Over the years, people have tried other foods or combinations to use for fast weight loss, and while there has been some success, it always comes back around to the potato taking center stage.

Resistant Starch

Early on in the establishment of the potato hack, I learned of resistant starch (RS). Resistant Starch is a special type of starch found in some starchy foods, i.e. corn, rice, bananas. The potato stands high above the rest in RS content, and RS has many tricks up its sleeve, as we'll talk about later. While I was researching RS, I became interested in the bacteria and fungi that grow in and on us. Collectively known as the "microbiome," this invisible life is vitally important to our wellbeing.

I have no doubt that there are other whole foods that could be used in a weight loss hack. On the top of my list are oats, yams, tiger nuts, and corn. These are the foods that sustained vast empires. All of these foods, and especially the potato, could be grown very easily and stored for long periods of time. Ironically, potatoes were one of the last foods discovered by humans as they marched out of Africa 4 million years ago. It even could be said that early humans stampeded around the globe in search of a perfect food such as the potato, and they found it...in the last place they looked.

Potassium and Sodium

The balance between potassium and sodium is almost universally skewed in favor of sodium when eating a diet filled with fast foods, processed foods, and snacks. This unfavorable balance is blamed for high blood pressure and heart disease. Reducing salt intake is one way to create a more favorable ratio, and increasing potassium is another. The problem is that sodium rich foods are everywhere in the standard American diet, while potassium rich foods take a bit more effort to find. What happens to this ratio during the potato hack?

The recommended daily allowance (RDA) of potassium set by the USDA is 4500mg per day. Three full pounds of potatoes has approximately 6000mg of potassium. This represents an intake that is 1/3 higher than the RDA for potassium. This RDA is the suggested intake level, not an upper limit of safety. With sodium, the RDA is no more than 2300mg. This represents an upper limit, quite different from the RDA for potassium. This indicates we need more potassium and less sodium.

In reality, surveys showed that only about 5% of us consume enough potassium and 13% eat less than the RDA of sodium. To recap:

Nutrient	Recommended	Actual
Sodium	Less than 2300mg	More than 3300mg
Potassium	More than 4500mg	Less than 2600mg

There is little danger of over-consuming potassium from real foods. Potassium supplements and potassium used as a salt substitute are seen as the most common cause of potassium overload. It's easy to google the dangers of too much potassium. The condition is called, hyperkalemia. This condition is seen in people with poor kidney function. It is not caused by eating potassium rich foods, though people with hyperkalemia are told to avoid potassium rich foods such as potatoes, tomatoes, oranges, and bananas. The most likely cause of hyperkalemia is from a reaction to certain medicines (ACE inhibitors, NSAIDs) or as a result of several diseases (i.e. Addison's Disease).

Potassium to Sodium Ratios while Potato Hacking

What is the ratio of sodium to potassium while potato hacking? It's hard to say. Calorie and nutrient calculators are all over the place. Some calculators show that eating 3-4 pounds of potatoes puts you in a "high sodium" category and others in "high potassium." This is because some nutrient calculators derive their figures based on how people normally eat the food, ie. skin off, heavily salted. Others show the nutrition figures based solely on the food itself, a sampling:

Source	Sodium	Potassium
CalorieKing	145mg (6%)	9979mg (212%)
FitDay	4609 (200%)	5752mg (122%)
NutritionData	175mg (8%)	9600mg (204%)
USDA	1068mg (46%)	3960mg (78%)

The general consensus is that potatoes are low in sodium and high in potassium, exactly as it should be for "proper balance." As it stands, there is NO vegetable in ANY amount that has a dangerously high level of potassium. If you have kidney problems and a medical condition that results in high potassium (hyperkalemia), or think you might, then consult with your doctor before trying the potato hack.

Potassium and sodium are two vital nutrients that play a big role in the success of the potato hack. I believe that when potato hacking, for the first time in most people's lives, their nutritional requirements are being fully met in a perfectly balanced way. Eating only potatoes for long periods of months or years could feasibly lead to some type of imbalance. Lots of smart people say otherwise, but to be on the safe side, let's keep the potato hack to 3-5 day increments and eat a well-balanced diet the rest of the time.

Alphabet Soup

Potatoes contain a plethora of micronutrients and chemicals that don't show up on the nutrition charts. They also affect a wide range of receptors in the body. When researchers start discussing these phytoalexins, steroids, receptors, and proteins we are generally greeted with blank stares and shuffling feet. We'll discuss these in-depth in the research chapter, but in case you skip it, here's the scoop.

Inside the potato we find KYNA, with its anti-inflammatory and neuroprotective abilities. Once in the gut, microbes turn potatoes into SCFA which fuels the immune system. Humans have several automatic systems to signal fullness or satiety. There is a hormone called CCK, that stimulates bile release and also suppresses hunger.

Then there is NYP, FFAR, POMV, CART, PYY, and GLP-1 to add to the list of hormones and enzymes that interact with potatoes. But the most powerful regulator of hunger is a *sore jaw* and a *full belly*.

The stretched-belly signals trump all the other signals. Possibly our modern excess of tasty, high-calorie foods have tempered the capacity of the "alphabet soup" of hunger hormones to do their job. After a meal of 2 pounds of potatoes, you will be DONE eating. So, the potato diet, in that regard, bypasses the need for a properly functioning set of hunger hormones and even helps to reset them.

To learn what all these alphabet soup acronyms mean, see the research chapter.

Satiety

Satiety refers to how "full" you feel after you eat. The old gag about feeling hungry soon after eating Chinese takeout may not be so farfetched when you look at the satiety levels of the foods involved. Researchers have long sought to learn what foods make us feel full and which leave us yearning for more. "Big Snacks," the makers of tasty junk food, spend considerable money and effort to sell us foods that keep us coming back for more.

The potato, however, is a food known for "sticking to your ribs." Holt et al. tested this hypothesis in 1995 and published the results in a paper, "The Satiety Index of Common Foods." They fed volunteers dozens of common foods and then compared how full they felt when compared to eating white bread. Potatoes were hands-down the big winner, but not any potato! French fries and potato chips scored lower than most foods, but the plain, boiled white potato loomed far above all other foods in terms of satiety.

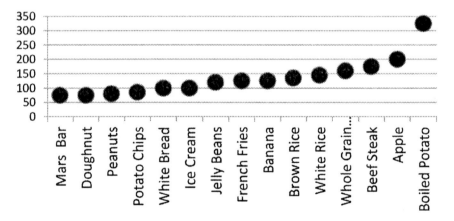

Satiety Index (Holt et al, 1995)

Nutrition Profile

Potatoes are a very nutritious food that can be prepared in a wide range of ways. The potato has undoubtedly contributed to the obesity epidemic the world is experiencing. When made into French fries, potato chips, and tater tots, it stops becoming a healthy food and turns into junk food. When potatoes are fried, they absorb large amounts of oil. Salted heavily and treated with preservatives, colors, and flavors, Americans are eating almost all of their potatoes in snack or fast food forms. According to the USDA potatoes account for 30% of all of the vegetables eaten in America, but only 9% are eaten as freshly prepared potatoes.

Nutrition Facts

Serving Size 1 potato (148g/5.3oz)

Amount Per Serving

Calories 110   Calories from Fat 0

	% Daily Value*
Total Fat 0g	0%
Saturated Fat 0g	0%
Trans Fat 0g	
Cholesterol 0mg	0%
Sodium 0mg	0%
Potassium 620mg	18%
Total Carbohydrate 26g	9%
Dietary Fiber 2g	8%
Sugars 1g	
Protein 3g	

Vitamin A 0%	•	Vitamin C 45%
Calcium 2%	•	Iron 6%
Thiamin 8%	•	Riboflavin 2%
Niacin 8%	•	Vitamin B_6 10%
Folate 6%	•	Phosphorous 6%
Zinc 2%	•	Magnesium 6%
Copper 4%		

*Percent Daily Values are based on a 2,000 calorie diet. Your daily values may be higher or lower depending on your calorie needs.

	Calories:	2,000	2,500
Total Fat	Less than	65g	80g
Sat Fat	Less than	20g	25g
Cholesterol	Less than	300mg	300mg
Sodium	Less than	2,400mg	2,400mg
Potassium		3,500mg	3,500mg
Total Carbohydrate		300g	375g
Dietary Fiber		25g	30g

As a standalone food, the potato is very nutritious. One medium potato contains 45% of the daily value for vitamin C and has more potassium than spinach, bananas, or broccoli. You can get 10% of your vitamin B6 from a medium potato. Potatoes are nearly fat free and contain no cholesterol. In addition to many other vitamins and minerals, potatoes contain a wide range of proteins. In fact, the same proteins found in the best grass-fed beef steak. Several official reports list the potato as having the best cost to nutrition ratio of any supermarket fruit or vegetable.

The source of all world knowledge, Wikipedia, hails the potato as a nutritional powerhouse:

> The potato contains vitamins and minerals, as well as an assortment of phytochemicals, such as carotenoids and natural phenols. Chlorogenic acid constitutes up to 90% of the potato tuber natural phenols. Others found in potatoes are 4-O-caffeoylquinic acid (crypto-chlorogenic acid), 5-O-caffeoylquinic (neo-chlorogenic acid), 3,4-dicaffeoylquinic and 3,5-dicaffeoylquinic acids. A medium-size 150 g (5.3 oz) potato with the skin provides 27 mg of vitamin C (45% of the Daily Value (DV)), 620 mg of potassium (18% of DV), 0.2 mg vitamin B6 (10% of DV) and trace amounts of thiamin, riboflavin, folate, niacin, magnesium, phosphorus, iron, and zinc (Wikipedia, 2015).

Keep in mind; these facts and figures all represent *one medium potato*. During the potato hack, we will be eating 10 or more medium potatoes a day! If you need a reference, a "medium potato" is about the size of a tennis ball. Next time you are at the supermarket, play around in the produce aisle weighing different sized potatoes to get a feel for what they weigh. These "mediums" generally go three-to-the-pound. A great big potato can weigh in at over a pound, but some have been known to weigh upwards of five pounds!

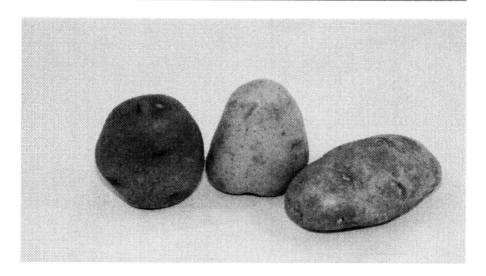

On a day of potatoes only, with four pounds eaten, the nutrition profile changes considerably. I've played around with nutrition calculators, and during a day on the potato hack, most people will be eating better than they have in years. Our modern taste for processed foods and their artificial flavors and colors are often fortified with minerals and vitamins. This fortification program is completely skewing our nutrient intake and filling us with unnatural sources of these vitamins and minerals. Here is a chart showing the percentages of recommended daily allowances of several key nutrients:

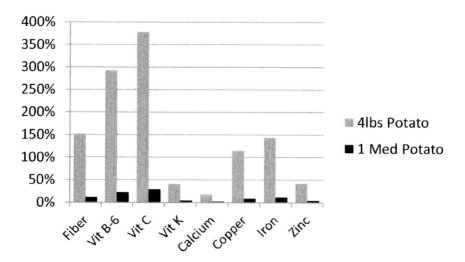

As you see, the nutritional profile of a medium potato is nothing like what we get on a full day of potato hacking. Calorie for calorie, even a ribeye steak is not as nutritionally balanced as the potato. Many people are concerned that a vegetarian diet does not deliver enough protein. While I agree that we need quality protein in our diets, does it need to come from meat? Let's look at the protein content of the potato.

Potato Protein Power

Protein is comprised of amino acids. For health purposes, there are nine "essential" amino acids that we must get through our diet. These essential amino acids are: histidine, isoleucine, leucine, lysine, methionine, phenylalanine, threonine, tryptophan, and valine. There are non-essential amino acids as well. Here is a look at the essential amino acids found in a potato:

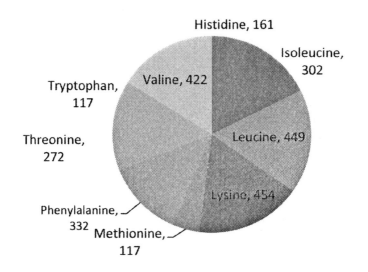

Note the presence of all nine essential amino acids. There are nine others as well. This is considered a "complete" amino acid score. In fact, the quality of proteins found in potatoes is better than that found in some meat and meat products. An all-potato diet will not leave you deficient in essential amino acids, and may in fact, be a diet higher in quality proteins than you are accustomed.

For the "gram counters," four pounds of potatoes contain 1400 calories with 37g of protein. A bit less than the recommended 40-60g from our government, but quite enough to get you through the day.

Pound-for-pound, calorie-for-calorie, potatoes are a nutritional powerhouse when looked at in terms of recommended daily allowances, but as you'll learn, there's even more to the potato than the government's RDAs. Potatoes hold secrets that are only now coming to light.

GMO Status

Potatoes are generally free from the ravages of pests and frost that prompted biotech labs to produce genetically modified corn, soybeans, and other commercial crops. However, potatoes are not immune to tinkering from scientists.

There are currently no Genetically Modified Organism (GMO) potatoes that you will find in a supermarket or farmer's market. There are a few GMO potato breeds being grown for industrial starch and chemical production. However, this is subject to rapid change. If you are against GMO foods in your diet, choose organically grown potatoes or grow your own. Thanks to a recent Whitehouse decision, GMO foods do not have to be labeled. Organic foods, on the other hand, cannot be from GMO seeds. Therefore, to avoid GMO foods, buy organic.

As a biotechnology major, I should have an opinion on GMO foods, but I'm torn. The science says there is nothing wrong with eating GMO foods, but I also know they have not been tested thoroughly. At this point, it is nearly impossible to avoid GMO foods in America. If you eat anything that comes in a wrapper, you are eating GMO foods.

Solanine, Chaconine, and Nightshade Sensitivity

Eating the leaves, vines, sprouts, and green spots of the potato can *kill*. Potatoes must have learned early in their evolution that insects and animals love their delicious underground tubers. Throughout the millennia, the potato perfected ways to protect itself. Potatoes belong to the *Solanacea* family of plants. Referred to as "nightshades," other members of this family include tomatoes, peppers (hot and sweet), eggplant, pimento, tomatillo, and tobacco. Nightshade sensitivity is an allergy to the proteins or alkaloids found in *Solanacea's* plants.

Glycoalkawhatsits?

Technically known as "glycoalkaloids α-solanine and α-chaconine," these natural plant steroids are indeed troubling. An examination of solanine and chaconine should scare us off from eating nightshades.

> *An acetylcholinesterase inhibitor (often abbreviated AChEI) or anti-cholinesterase, is a chemical or a drug that inhibits the acetylcholinesterase enzyme from breaking down acetylcholine, thereby increasing both the level and duration of action of the neurotransmitter acetylcholine.*

In commercially available potatoes, the solanine content is required by law to be less than 20 milligrams (mg) per kilogram (kg). At this level, it is considered non-toxic; however, the solanine can accumulate in green spots and eyes. The National Institute of Environmental Health Sciences determined that the average consumption of solanine and other potato toxins was 12.75 mg per person per day, and that the lowest dose that showed toxic effects in humans is 5 times that at 1mg per kg of body-weight, or about 50-70mg per day (Tice, Chaconine and Solanine; Review of Toxicological Literature, 1998). Some estimate that you'd have to eat two pounds of fully green potatoes to receive a fatal dose of solanine and chaconine.

A day of potato hacking, at the extreme upper end with five full pounds of potato, could mean ingesting approximately 40mg of glycoalkaloids. This is below the threshold shown to produce toxicity. These glycoalkaloids are concentrated in the skins of potatoes, so carefully removing all hints of green from each potato is recommended. The danger of ingesting green potatoes needs to be emphasized, there have been several documented cases of potato poisoning, such as:

> *McMillan and Thompson (1979) reported a poisoning incident involving 78 adolescent boys attending a U.K. school, who became ill after eating a batch of potatoes that had been left in stores over the summer term. Seventeen (22%) of the boys who ate the potatoes were hospitalized*

> *with symptoms of vomiting, severe diarrhea, abdominal pain,*
> *fever, hallucinations and other nervous system effects. The*
> *three most critically ill were comatose or stuporose and had*
> *peripheral circulatory collapse at the time of hospital admis-*
> *sion. The glycoalkaloid content of the potatoes was measured*
> *as 0.25 to 0.3 mg/g peeled, boiled potato (Tice, 1998).*

A standard warning needs to apply. Signs of solanine/chaconine toxicity are burning and tingling lips and throat immediately after consuming, and diarrhea, nausea, and gastrointestinal distress within a few hours. Solanine does not accumulate readily in the body and is eliminated in approximately 12 hours by the healthy human. Solanine and chaconine are found in very high levels in French fries and potato chips, yet you never hear of anyone getting sick from these common sources and there certainly are no warnings at fast-food joints that "French fries may kill!"

$$ Here's a million-dollar idea for someone…write a diet book called *Potatoes: The Root of all Health Problems*, or *Spud Butt*, something catchy. In this book, discuss acetylcholinesterase inhibitors, nightshades, and glycoalkaloids. Tell people that if they avoid all potatoes, they will see better health. Guess what? It will work! But not because of the "poisons" found in potatoes, but because of the lower amounts of cooking oils and processed snacks in their diet.

If you feel you may have been poisoned by potatoes, get to the emergency room and bring some of the potatoes you ate. Treatments include IV fluids and anticonvulsant medicines. Often potato poisoning is mistreated as a viral or bacterial infection. A reliable method to test for extremely high levels of solanine and chaconine is to simply place a bit of the raw potato to your lips. If you feel tingling and burning, the potato is not safe to eat.

It is my sincere hope that no one discovers they have a nightshade allergy when they first try the potato hack. Surely anyone with a nightshade allergy has known of their condition through previous exposure to nightshades.

Acrylamide

When starchy foods are browned during cooking, called the "Maillard reaction," some of them form a chemical called acrylamide. Acrylamide is used in many industrial applications, in fact over 300 million pounds are produced and sold in the US alone. Acrylamide is considered a carcinogen.

In 2002, scientists found high levels of acrylamide in potato chips and French fries. This prompted a health scare that these foods would cause cancer. Many, many research studies were performed to determine if food-based acrylamides were the source of the explosion in cancer cases around the world. Fourteen years later, there is no consensus.

Humans have consumed heated starches for many thousands of years, speculation abounds that possibly humans have adapted to the ingestion of dietary acrylamides. The World Health Orgaization (WHO), FDA, and governments around the world have all issued weakly worded warnings against the consumption of high-acrylamide foods. If acrylamide is a concern of yours, simply avoid potato chips and French fries…two foods not allowed on the potato hack anyway.

Prebiotic and Probiotic!

The holy grail of gut health and good digestion is the right combination of microbes and the proper food to feed them. The fact that our guts are colonized by trillions of bacteria that effect our health is not just speculation anymore. In fact, the need for a properly functioning microbiome has spurred a multi-billion-dollar industry of probiotic pills and prebiotic fibers available for consumer purchase.

With the potato hack, you get the best of both worlds. Potatoes contain resistant starch, an established prebiotic fiber that feeds predominantly the beneficial bacteria in your intestines. What most people do not realize, potatoes also contain a complement of microbial life that reside deep within the potato itself.

It was long thought that all bacteria associated with plants was found clinging to the surface. Recent studies show that potatoes and other plants contain "endophytic" bacteria and fungi. These endophytes are there to help the potato grow and defend itself against invaders. However, the potato shares these endophytes with you when you eat it, providing you with their DNA, microRNA, and healthy enzymes. Our immune system gets a boost when it sees these hidden bacteria and fungi as well.

To Peel or Not to Peel?

In light of the "potato poison" situation, is it best to peel all of your potatoes when potato hacking? Possibly, but not just because of possible glycoalkaloids present. Potatoes are one of the most important food items in the world. Billions of tons are bought and sold around the globe every year. One of the qualities of potatoes that make them such a valuable commodity is their staying power.

Commercial potatoes have bigger problems than their natural plant chemicals. Potatoes are sprayed in the field with herbicides and pesticides. A potato can be stored for well over a year without any sign of greening or sprouting. This requires the use of antifungals and sprout inhibitors. By the time a potato gets to the supermarket, it's been kept in an artificial environment and bathed in chemicals.

Luckily, most of these chemicals are found only in the peel. Peeling a potato can be a good way to prevent exposure to unwanted agricultural toxins. With this in mind, I always peel <u>supermarket</u> potatoes. When it comes to organic potatoes, which hopefully were not treated with chemicals, I only peel them if they look unappetizing, i.e. black spots, green spots, sprouts, cuts, bruises. The same goes for my homegrown potatoes. Which would you prefer?

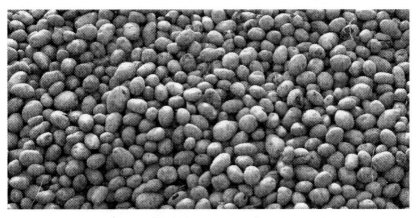

Commercially Grown Potatoes (Pixabay.com)

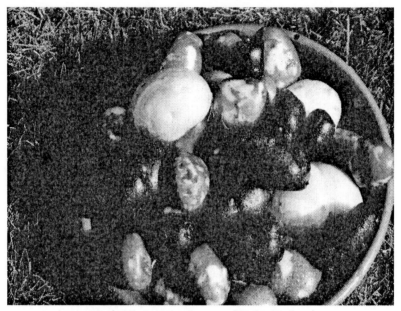

Tim's Homegrown Potatoes (Author's Photo)

Wrap-up

Potatoes are good food. Humans have been eating them for thousands of years. Very few cases of potato poisoning exist when compared to the prodigious amount of potatoes consumed. Sports bars all over America have absolutely no qualms in selling tons of potato peels to their customers. I've yet to hear of a case where people were poisoned eating potato chips, French fries, stuffed potato peels, or any other incantation of potato products

Potatoes are a great source of nutrients. Pound-for-pound, one of the cheapest as well. If you've eaten potatoes your whole life without issues, you won't have a problem doing the potato hack. Potatoes are *food;* standard food safe-practices and common sense must be applied. Remove any signs of green and sprouts. Peel at your own discretion.

For the purposes of the "potato" hack, we'll stick with potatoes. If anyone wants to try an oat, tiger nut, or corn hack, I'd love to read your book. Just be prepared for the question: "Can I use potatoes instead?"

POTATO QUOTES

"I APPRECIATE THE POTATO ONLY AS A PROTECTION AGAINST FAMINE, EXCEPT FOR THAT, I KNOW OF NOTHING MORE EMINENTLY TASTELESS."

Anthelme Brillat-Savarin (1755-1826)
'The Physiology of Taste' (1825)

Notes:

Chapter 7. Potato Hack Icons

Dr. Chris Voigt

In 2010, Chris Voigt, head of the Washington State Potato Commission, ate a potato-only diet for 60 days. He did this to promote potatoes as a nutritious, cost-effective food at a time when the USDA was revising its stance on the inclusion of the potato in school lunches and other social programs.

> *This is not the new fad diet. It was really to make a bold statement, to remind people that the potato is truly healthy and nutritious (Voigt, TODAY, 2010)*

Indeed, the potato hack is not meant to be a "fad diet" either, but a way of using a common, nutritious food to reset our metabolism, lose some weight, and then get on with life, free from diet plans and constant worrying about what we eat. Dr. Voigt did not *quite* follow the rules of the potato hack he helped inspire, but he's still an inspiration, no?

> *No toppings, no sour cream, no butter. It was literally just potatoes and seasoning, and oil for cooking (Voigt, TODAY, 2010)*

With the exception of cooking oil, Voigt did justice to the 1849 potato diet. His results were a drop in 21 pounds in weight, and 67 points of LDL cholesterol.

> *Physically I feel great. Lots of energy, sleep good at night, no strange side-effects. I'm not encouraging anyone to go on this crazy diet, nor would my doctor. This diet was just a bold statement to remind people that there is a lot of nutrition in a potato. (Voigt, BBC News, 2010)*

Dr. Voigt's hopes were that this diet would generate some publicity for the lowly potato. Potatoes have been greatly maligned by the dieting world as an "empty carb." Unfortunately, the USDA also bought into this misnomer.

> *If we are successful in convincing USDA to put potatoes in the programs, then I'd call it a 100 percent success. But it's been great that the publicity and the general awareness the public has now and how it's drawn some attention to the nutritional value of potatoes. I just consider that gravy (Voigt, TODAY, 2010).*

And Voigt was successful! First, in 2011, Congress overturned a motion to limit potatoes from school lunches. Then, in December, 2014, the USDA issued a memorandum: "Eligibility of White Potatoes for Purchase with the Cash – Value Voucher." According to the memo, potatoes would be allowed for purchase with WIC cash vouchers. WIC (Women, Infants, Children) gives needy pregnant women and mothers government-subsidized vouchers to buy nutritious food for their family. To exclude the potato from such a program is mind-boggling.

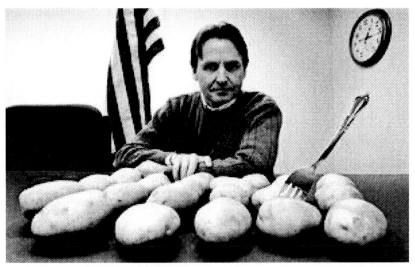

Kudos to Dr. Chris Voigt for sparking a potato revolution (Seattle Times).

Scottish Prisoners of 1840

Throughout history, people have survived—and thrived—on a diet consisting wholly of potatoes. Criminals in prisons were often fed only potatoes and thrived. Here is a blast from the past you will enjoy, and you will soon agree that these Scottish prisoners deserve their place on this honor roll. Please keep in mind as you read this account of experimental diets for prisoners that weight loss was NOT the goal. Overall health and satisfaction were the desired outcomes.

"Fifth Report of the Inspectors of Prisons of Scotland," by Frederick Hill, 1840.

> *During the present year, an experiment in diet has been made in the Glasgow Bridewell [prison], which, although not carried on for a sufficient time, and under a sufficient variety of circumstances, to render it safe to adopt as a guide, appears to me to be of sufficient interest and importance to record, and to submit to your lordship's attention (Hill, 1840).*

The prison management embarked on an experiment to find an optimal diet for their charges. They devised eight different diets and fed these diets to different groups of prisoners for a month at a time. The diets were combinations of meat, potatoes, oatmeal, and milk. Without exception, the favored diet was the all-potato diet. Keep in mind, the goal was adequate nutrition, not weight loss. The prisoners were each given 6 pounds of potatoes, split into three meals. The potatoes were all boiled, and presumably served hot. Ironically, several of the experimental diets used baked potatoes, which were abjectly rejected by all prisoners.

Ordinary prison diet

- Breakfast—Eight ounces of oatmeal, made into porridge with a pint of buttermilk.

- Dinner—Two pints of broth, containing four ounces of barley and one ounce of bone, with vegetables; also eight ounces of bread.

- Supper—Five ounces of oatmeal, made into porridge, with half a pint of buttermilk.

The All-Potato Diet

- Breakfast—Two pounds of potatoes, boiled.
- Dinner—Three pounds of potatoes, boiled.
- Supper—One pound of potatoes, boiled.

> *A class of ten young men and boys was put on this diet. All had been in confinement for short periods only, and all were employed at light work, teasing [working with horse hair]. At the beginning of the experiment eight were in good health and two in indifferent health; at the end, the eight continued in good health, and the two who had been in indifferent health had improved. There was, on an average, a gain in weight of nearly three and a half pounds per prisoner, the greatest gain being eight and a quarter pounds, by a young man, whose health had been indifferent at the beginning of the experiment. Only two prisoners lost at all in weight, and the quantity in each case was trifling. The pris-*

oners all expressed themselves quite satisfied with this diet, and regretted the change back again to the ordinary diet.

Normally when we think of "punishment food," we think of bread and water. The Uniform Code of Military Justice still has provisions for putting naughty soldiers on "limited rations," which in the old days meant bread and water. The US Prison System has taken "bread and water" to a whole new level.

In prisons across the country, unruly prisoners are fed "nutraloaf." This fruitcake-like concoction is a doughy food substitute that contains all the calories and nutrients a prisoner needs to live. Prisoners complain when fed nutraloaf, unlike the potato-fed prisoners of old.

Antoine Augustin Parmentier (1737-1813)

Parmentier is a familiar name in potato circles. Many potato dishes are named in his honor. A French scholar, he's credited with bringing potatoes into cultivation in Europe and the subsequent population explosion the potato enabled. Antoine Parmentier is also one of the first people to embrace the potato hack.

As a prisoner of the Seven Years' War (1754-1763), Parmentier was fed nothing but potatoes for weeks at a stretch. At this time, potatoes were not seen as human food, but used for feeding livestock. Parmentier's Prussian guards certainly got a chuckle out of feeding prisoners animal fodder. Parmentier got the last laugh.

Trained as a nutritionist and pharmacist, Parmentier noticed right away that prisoners being fed potatoes were thriving. Parmentier, having no preconceptions about the newly introduced European potatoes, remarked that he quite enjoyed the meals of potato mash. While imprisoned, Parmentier schemed ways in which the potato could be commercially grown and used to solve the growing food crisis in France.

After the war, Parmentier gained notoriety by throwing lavish dinner parties where the only thing on the menu was *pomme de terre*. Considered poisonous by most Frenchmen, Parmentier had an uphill battle. Of course, he knew the views held by his countrymen were laughable after his treatment in the Prussian prisons.

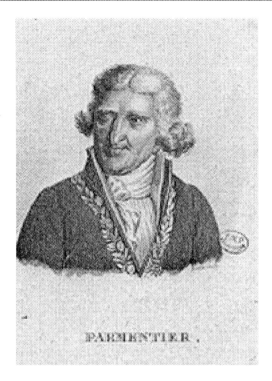

PARMENTIER.

Anonymous Potato Hackers

Over the years, I've talked with hundreds of people in various forums about the potato hack. Using fake usernames or just "anonymous," these are the people that kept me interested in proselytizing the virtues of the potato hack.

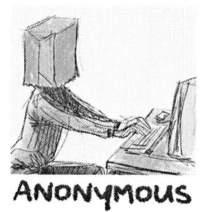

ANONYMOUS

❝ Hey all – Just starting my first PH (day 3). Loving it. Using just salt. I have very good discipline in general, once I believe in what I am doing.

Over the years (I'm 55), I've done extended water fasts, juice fasts, mono-diets, rotation diets, vegan, Atkins, VLC, super-paleo, super-foods, etc. (I've resolved very serious health issues through diet hacking – different hacks added to body knowledge and addressed different issues – and my health is now very strong – much better in most ways than at any time in my 30s and 40s)... Compared to all those interventions, PH is easy and very comforting.

I'm thrilled to have found it, and very excited to experiment further. Wish I had found it earlier. Not much discipline required at all. I suspect that most of the trouble people have doing it (keeping the rules), is all mental/emotional/habitual. The body response seems very natural and effortless, and even pleasant – at least so far.

Thanks to Tim and all for your research and sharing! It is an exciting time we are living in, with the access to information and rapid pace of health knowledge expansion (Anonymous, Potato Hack Blog, Dec 2015).

❝ I don't understand why everyone seems so keen to modify what is clearly a simple, effective, and may I say even elegant hack.

Stuffing down potatoes 'til you barf, adding in fat free miracle whip – are we getting trolls in here or are people really just so unable to control themselves?

Not only are potatoes, by themselves, the perfect food for this for many reasons. Tim has, if you're paying attention, explained, the other benefit to this hack is that it introduces some self-discipline. Let's face it, in an awful lot of cases it's lack of self-discipline that caused the unwanted weight gain and subsequent health difficulties to begin with (Anonymous, Potato Hack Blog, Dec 2015).

❝ Wow. Straight Potato Diet since the 1st of November. Figuring to finish out the week on only potatoes. Started the first by fasting until supper time, then only potatoes since. I have been eating only boiled (Russet, Yukon, and Red) potatoes with salt and spice for lunch and supper. I started at 206.8 lbs. on Sunday morning, and this morning I weighed 201.6 lbs. Figuring to finish on Friday and eat something else on Saturday and Sunday. I may start again on next Monday, we'll see.

I'm amazed at the weight loss. I've been plant-based for 4 months and had lost 18 lbs., but was stalled and a few bad habits had crept in. This has been a great reset and jump-start at the same time to get me off the plateau where I had found myself not able to get off the 205ish for a while.

Loving this. Honestly, the potatoes still taste good to me. I usually do just plain, cold, boiled reds for lunch, then for supper I cut the boiled russets into fries and then just bake them to crispy and eat with malt vinegar (per your suggestion, thank you). Tastes great every time.

This is great! ("jss," Potato Hack Blog, Nov 2015).

Just lost 15 pounds. Took me a little bit to believe it was easier just to just follow your strict rules. For me, I eat boiled, cooled potatoes for lunch and for dinner M-F Saturday and Sunday I eat a nutrient dense diet including leaner grass-fed meat, liver, eggs, vegetables, rice and all the fruit I want. Last weekend I had buckwheat pancakes for breakfast one day and fermented oatmeal porridge the next day. When I am satisfied I stop eating. I really like this diet. I eat my satiating potatoes for the week I am at work and it is so easy to forgo all the doughnuts and treats that are a regular part of the office. I just know M-F it is potatoes. I don't tired or hungry. I have plenty of energy. So much easier and comfortable than HCG or ketosis. When I was low-carbing I had so many problems with sleep. Now, I can't stay awake even if I want to! I don't have to wear orange glasses or stay away from screens. Thank-you. Thank-you! ("AH", Potato Hack Blog, Nov 2014).

This potato diet is really bothering me. It works 'too well', that is, I can't understand it(!)

I've read all the posited explanations here and on other blogs last year, but when I do it and vary one parameter at a time, protein or fat, I still am no closer to a clue as to what's really happening because nothing is explaining the original mystery: the weight loss at low fat-protein amounts even for 1200kC worth of potatoes is as if I ate NOTHING the previous day. Zip. No calories.

Here's what I've got so far:

- 3-4 lbs a day of boiled or microwaved potatoes, as long as using only 1T of fat per 2lbs, always give me about 0.6-0.7lbs loss daily. It's as if I ate nothing at all (my daily reqs are only about 1800kC).
- Add up to 2T of fat per 2 lbs potatoes, get less weight loss but still about 0.4 lbs loss per day.
- Above 2T it shuts off on me, no loss.
- Add 7-10gms protein (eg. ham, minced meat, even liver) to each 2 lb meal, same large 0.6-0.7lbs loss.
- Add more than that protein, loss moderates kinda linearly, until I can't detect it anymore at around 40gms protein a day.

It isn't water loss, none of it. Impedance scales are useless for absolute numbers but relative numbers are fine – no change day to day. Plus, none of the usual changes you get on dehydration or on starting a ketogenic diet (urine color, skin suppleness, water consumption/frequency...). Of course, it's not expected either, since gorging on starch/glucose in potatoes so plenty of glycogen. But hey, nothing else about this works as expected, so I made sure to check the hydration state.

Anyone have similar observations re. unexplainable large weight loss? ("EpiCurie," Mark's Daily Apple Nutrition Forum, October 2013).

I'm down another two pounds; that is 12 pounds in 2 1/2 weeks. I still feel very comfortable and am not craving anything.

Very impressive hack! ("KT," Low Carb Friends Forum, February 2013).

I think the potato hack has already proven itself successful for most people and it's worth taking seriously, so hopefully we can concentrate a bit more on the how and why, rather than "if". Maybe even some recipes.

Tried the PPD twice now, both times lost a couple of pounds (as net loss, despite some mild regaining later). I stick to no more than 3 or 4 days though, as I find it hard to believe there's really enough protein and I'm not getting any fat-soluble vitamins etc. Besides, I now live in Malaysia and this place is very into the whole eating out with the family thing.

Others seem happy going 2 weeks so why not? ("AC," Mark's Daily Apple Nutrition Forum, November 2012).

And of course, "this guy:"

❝Can't I just use eggs, or cheese, or bananas? ("Anon," Mark's Daily Apple Nutrition Forum, May 2012).

Well deserving of honor are the Potato Hackers I've chatted with over the past several years on various internet platforms.

Matt Damon

Matt Damon stars in the 2015 Hollywood movie, *The Martian,* based on Andy Weir's 2011 novel by the same name. Matt Damon plays an American astronaut stranded on Mars in the year 2035.

Alone and starving, astronaut Mark Watney (played by Damon) remembers that the Mars research lab is stocked with potatoes that the crew had brought along for their first Thanksgiving in space. Using his own "waste" as fertilizer, Watney grows an impressive crop of potatoes and survives by eating them for 459 "sols."

I was quite touched with the movie. Matt Damon went through all the stages of grief when he found he was stranded alone on Mars. First he was in denial, surely they did not just abandon him on Mars! Then he was angry. Moping around for sols on end while he ate through his food supply. He threw temper fits and cursed like a madman. Then he bargained that Mars would not beat him as he used all his NASA training to become the "best botanist on Mars!" Eventually, Damon's character accepted his fate and *just ate his potatoes.*

And so it is with the potato hack. It's amusing how people react when they first learn of the potato hack. Denial, anger, bargaining, and acceptance. Never fails. People always say, "Won't work for me!" Then they become angry because they are firmly attached to their present diet, even if it is not working. People actually get mad at me. How dare I propose such a radical plan, it must be flawed! But then they try it. They do the potato hack, lose a bunch of weight, find they are not starving, and *just eat their potatoes.*

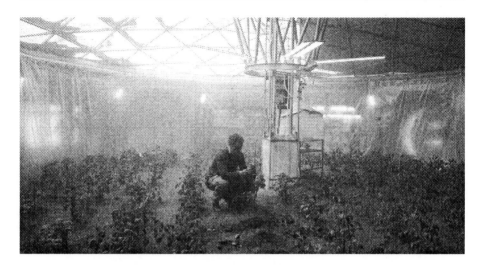

Matt Damon; First Potato Hacker on Mars! (20th Century Fox)

POTATO QUOTES

"I'LL SPEND THE REST OF THE EVENING ENJOYING A POTATO. AND BY "ENJOYING" I MEAN "HATING SO MUCH I WANT TO KILL PEOPLE."

— *MARK WATNEY, THE MARTIAN (2014)*

Notes:

Chapter 8. Inquiring Minds Only... Science!

To answer your most pressing question, yes, I realize that what I am saying seems incredible. I'm not the first person to present a mono-food diet. Most mono-food diets, such as the Grapefruit Diet, will lead to weight loss. "Eat this one weird food to bust belly fat!" I've seen them too. But the potato hack is different. The potato hack uses the natural pharmacological properties of S. *tuberosum* to exert physiological changes.

If potatoes were a drug, the preclinical studies were performed over the 10,000 years since the potato's discovery in the Andes mountains. Toxicity, pharmacokinetics, pharmacodynamics, formulation, and delivery systems have been tested by each group of people that were introduced to S. *tuberosum*. The French, being leery of the nightshade relationship, first only fed potatoes to animals. When the animals thrived, they tested it on prisoners of war, and then the poor.

Potato hack "trials" were completed throughout the 1700s and 1800s as millions of people subsisted on diets of just potatoes. Later trials were conducted over the years in which potatoes were fed to select groups of people in a hospital ward setting. These studies were largely ignored because there was no obesity epidemic (quite the opposite!) and drugs soon replaced food for diseases like cancer, diabetes, and high blood pressure.

The FDA does not regulate food used as drugs. If they did, potatoes would surely be outlawed due to their content of pharmaceutical grade glycoalkaloids and kynurenic acid (**KYNA**).

Discussion

In this chapter I will delve into scientific research. Throughout the book, I try to keep citations and references minimal for a better reading experience. This chapter will be heavy on citations with references to scholarly, peer-reviewed research journals. Please do explore the research and feel free to come to your own conclusions.

Having spent many years reading scientific papers, it's safe to say that for every paper one can find in support of an argument, an equal number can be found in disagreement. I try to present both sides, or stick with papers that simply show the underlying mechanisms of biology that make the potato hack what it is. Keep in mind that even though they pretend to, scientists don't know everything.

The holy grail of health is the prevention of inflammation. Systemic inflammation is seen to be the root of most health problems but pinning down the source of inflammation is difficult. Much of the potato hack's success is in the reduction of inflammation. There is also a theoretical "weight set-point." Many of the trademarked diets promise to lower your body's weight set-point, much like turning down the thermostat in your house. The potato hack is the only dieting strategy I have found that actually delivers on this promise of reducing inflammation and lowering the body's weight set-point.

The potato hack is an extreme low-fat dietary intervention. Low-fat diets have been used for decades to treat all manner of metabolic dysfunction. It's also a low-calorie diet in most cases. We'll explore the use of the "calories-in calories-out" model of weight loss. Insulin sensitivity is a great marker of health. The potato hack is very good at reversing the issues that cause metabolic syndrome in adults. As people lose their ability to handle dietary glucose, it starts a cascade of that leads to high cholesterol, high blood pressure, weight gain and other metabolic derangements.

Lately health science has shifted to a focus on the interactions of gut microbes in human health. There is a well-proven "brain-gut" connection in which microbial communities living within your intestines can exert influence on the "auto-pilot" systems in the brain. This brain-gut connection is a double-edged sword and with modern, processed foods, the brain-gut connection likely works against you. The potato hack resets the circuits. Additionally, we will explore the science behind "food reward" theories. Your brain plays tricks on your body when you eat a diet filled with non-stop tasty treats. The potato hack bypasses the reward centers in the brain and puts you firmly in control of your eating habits. The compounds that a potato produces to protect itself from frost and drought make it a virtual pharmacy.

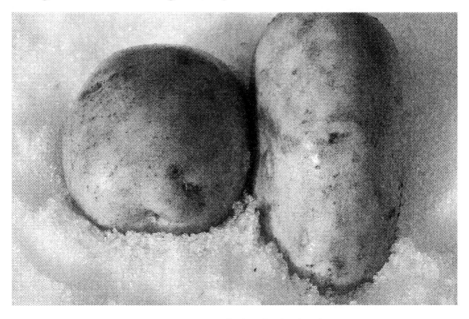

Snow Spuds (Author's Photo)

Finally, we'll take a look at some of the compounds and molecules found in potatoes that make them such a perfect food for a short-term dietary intervention. It you are a consummate skeptic like me, you'll enjoy reading along as I lay out the science behind the potato hack. If science bores you to death, feel free to skip this section entirely.

- Anti-Inflammatory
- Weight Set-point
- Low-fat
- Calories-in Calories-out
- Insulin Sensitivity
- Intestinal Microbiome, aka "Gut Biome," "Gut Flora,"
- Food Reward Theories

Anti-Inflammatory Actions of Potatoes

Kynurenic Acid

Kynurenic acid (KYNA) has been described in medical literature since 1853. KYNA is a metabolite of tryptophan which acts as an endogenous antagonist of ionotropic glutamate receptors [Sorry, I told you the science was heavy!]. KYNA plays an important role in the central nervous system and the brain. KYNA also exerts anti-inflammatory actions throughout the body, but especially in the gut. KYNA's anti-ulcerative and anti-hypermotility properties could prove useful in treating IBS and colitis. Additionally, KYNA has anti-cancer and antioxidant properties (Turski, 2012).

KYNA can be found in most foods eaten, but the highest amounts are in two foods long considered exceptionally healthful: honey and potatoes. Potatoes have 10 times as much KYNA as the next leading sources. It is thought that potatoes are the leading source of KYNA in the human body. Experiments with KYNA in the brain show that it is a very important for cognitive functions and is well regulated as it crosses the blood-brain barrier (Pocivavsek, 2011). KYNA's actions in the gut, however, are much more dependent on dietary intake and is possibly crucial for proper gut function (Turski, 2013).

Solanine/Chaconine

Earlier we discussed the potato glycoalkaloids, α – chaconine, α –solanine, two compounds found in potatoes that are normally associated with negative consequences. I mentioned that quite possibly there is more to the story than these secondary plant metabolites being inherently harmful. In fact, chaconine and solanine quite possibly are one of the leading anti-inflammatory factors that make the potato hack so special.

Kenny et al. (2013), explored the anti-inflammatory properties of the potato glycoalkaloids and determined that "...sub-cytotoxic concentrations of potato glycoalkaloids and potato peel extracts possess anti-inflammatory effects in vitro and with further investigation may be useful in the prevention of anti-inflammatory diseases." They examined the anti-inflammatory effects of potato glycoalkaloids using human and murine T cell models. This group of researchers were seeking to discover if potatoes had many of the same anti-inflammatory properties attributed to tomatoes, noting the similarities in tomato and potato glycoalkaloids.

This study presents novel findings that the glycoalkaloids present in potatoes are effective at managing pro-inflammatory cytokines and LPS induced inflammation. They found that the aglycone unit of glycoalkaloids is responsible for the anti-inflammatory action. Potato glycoalkaloids are "nitrogen analogues of steroid saponins, such as diosgenin, a compound that has proven effective in inhibiting inflammatory responses."

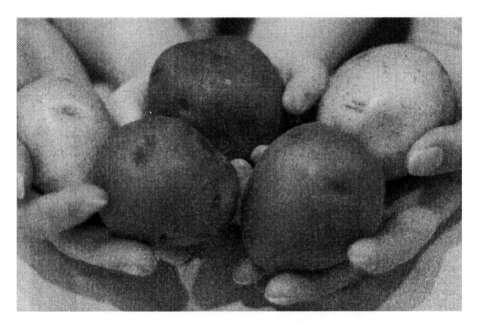

A 2014 study was conducted to examine the effects of solanine on pancreatic cancer. This research was a follow-up on earlier reports that solanine was effective against liver cancer and melanomas (Lv et al., 2014). The researchers discovered that solanine was effective at "suppressing the pathway proliferation, angiogenesis and metastasis" of pancreatic cancer. The main anti-cancer actions of solanine are believed to be due to effects of anti-inflammatory actions against interleukin-2 and 8 (Lv et al., 2014).

> In the present study, we used non-toxic concentration of α-Solanine(3, 6 and 9 µg/µl) and found that α-Solanine inhibits metastasis in vitro, such as invasion, migration and angiogenesis, indicating that the inhibitory effect of α-Solanine on metastasis was not by its cytotoxic function. We first evaluated the efficacy

of α-Solanine in vivo and found α-Solanine can inhibit proliferation, angiogenesis and metastasis in tumor xenograft in athymic nude mice.

I think that it is important to note that this study used non-lethal doses, indicating that the beneficial effects of the potato hack are real. Rarely do people eat potatoes to the exclusion of all other foods. Solanine has a 12 hour life in the human body, being readily excreted in the urine (Dolan, 2010). A sustained feeding of potatoes as with the potato hack undoubtedly exudes anti-inflammatory processes within the body.

Building on the work of Kenny (2013) and Lv (2014), a paper in the Journal of Agriculture and Food Chemistry analyzed the chemistry and anti-cancer mechanisms of potato glycoalkaloids (Friedman, 2015). Friedman discusses the anti-cancer and anti-tumor effects seen in vivo and in vitro associated with potato glycoalkaloids.

Showing many activities of potato glycoalkaloids against various forms of cancer, Friedman (2015) states, "With respect to potatoes, unofficial worldwide guidelines recommend a guideline for total glycoalkaloid content of 20 mg/100 g fresh weight. On the basis of the anticarcinogenic results discussed earlier, it seems that this level in commercial potatoes might help to protect against multiple cancers."

Another group also explored the anti-inflammatory effects of potatoes in 2015. Using potato peel extract, Xu et al. demonstrated pharmacological activities of potato glycoalkaloids on COPD from smoking.

> When pro-inflammatory cytokines were activated, oxygen-free radicals and lysosomal enzymes were always released by these neutrophils causing inflammation. The reduced expression of G-CSF by PE [potato peel extract] further illustrated that the inflammatory process in COPD was relieved. To sum up, we suspect PE was able to relieve inflammation of lung tissue by inhibiting TNF-α and G-CSF, activating IL-10, and thereby effectively treating CS [cigarette smoke]-induced COPD.

Potato peel extracts contains amino acids, vitamins, minerals, and organics. Potatoes are effective in anti-inflammation. The amino acids and vitamins found in potatoes only exhibit secondary effects on inflammation and not direct anti-inflammatory effects.

Not only anti-inflammatory, but anti-cancer as well. Could it be that the very chemicals we were taught to fear in high doses are the best thing about the potato hack? If solanine and chaconine are indeed anti-inflammatory as the research suggests, the potato hack is the ultimate elimination diet. A few days on a restricted potato diet to reduce inflammation and then a gradual reintroduction of normal foods to see which are causing inflammation. Additionally, those on chemotherapy for cancer are often told to reduce carbs in their diet (LaGory, 2013). This advice should not apply to anticarcinogenic potatoes. Furthermore, as we've seen with resveratrol extract and other wonder drugs, it will undoubtedly come to pass that the real "magic" is in whole potatoes and not some extract. The potato hack provides a massive, yet sub-toxic, dose of all the anti-inflammatory glycoalakaloids in their whole form.

References:

Dolan, L. C., Matulka, R. A., & Burdock, G. A. (2010). Naturally occurring food toxins. *Toxins, 2*(9), 2289-2332.

Friedman, M. (2015). Chemistry and Anticarcinogenic Mechanisms of Glycoalkaloids Produced by Eggplants, Potatoes, and Tomatoes. *Journal of agricultural and food chemistry, 63*(13), 3323-3337.

Kenny, O. M., McCarthy, C. M., Brunton, N. P., Hossain, M. B., Rai, D. K., Collins, S. G., ... & O'Brien, N. M. (2013). Anti-inflammatory properties of potato glycoalkaloids in stimulated Jurkat and Raw 264.7 mouse macrophages. *Life sciences, 92*(13), 775-782.

LaGory, E. L., & Giaccia, A. J. (2013). A low-carb diet kills tumor cells with a mutant p53 tumor suppressor gene: The Atkins diet suppresses tumor growth. *Cell Cycle, 12*(5), 718-719.

Lv, C., Kong, H., Dong, G., Liu, L., Tong, K., Sun, H., ... & Zhou, M. (2014). Antitumor efficacy of á-solanine against pancreatic cancer in vitro and in vivo. *PloS one, 9*(2), e87868.

Pocivavsek, A., Wu, H. Q., Potter, M. C., Elmer, G. I., Pellicciari, R., & Schwarcz, R. (2011). Fluctuations in endogenous kynurenic acid control hippocampal glutamate and memory. *Neuropsychopharmacology, 36*(11), 2357-2367.

Turski, M. P., Kamiński, P., Zgrajka, W., Turska, M., & Turski, W. A. (2012). Potato-an important source of nutritional kynurenic acid. *Plant foods for human nutrition, 67*(1), 17-23.

Turski, M. P., Turska, M., Paluszkiewicz, P., Parada-Turska, J., & Oxenkrug, G. F. (2013). Kynurenic Acid in the Digestive system—new Facts, new challenges. *International journal of tryptophan research: IJTR, 6*, 47.

Xu, G. H., Shen, J., Sun, P., Yang, M. L., Zhao, P. W., Niu, Y., … & Liu, L. L. (2015). Anti-inflammatory effects of potato extract…

Weight Set-point

Weight set-point theories get bounced around in the main stream media from time-to-time. Nearly every diet promises a reset of your weight set-point. But few realize what the weight set-point really is and how it can be effectively lowered. Humans have built-in feedback mechanisms to keep their body weight fairly constant year-round. We should all strive to keep our weight within a 5 to10-pound band from year to year, being careful not to begin the steady increase in weight that results in obesity.

Weight set-point theory revolves around our body's ability to sense body weight and raise or lower it with hunger signals, increased metabolism, hormonal changes, or desire for certain nutrients (Harris, 1990). The end-goal being a body in equilibrium by regulating weight. The weight at which the body settles is not thought to be easily manipulated.

Many scientists believe that the weight set-point is largely inherited and hard to change, influenced also by the modern food supply in which high calorie foods are continually available. In the Minnesota starvation study, healthy controls were starved for 24 weeks, then allowed to eat ad libitum. During starvation, people lost an average of 66% of their fat mass, and upon re-feeding they added fat back on to 145% of their pre-starvation weight, dubbed "catch-up fat phenomenon (DeAndrade, 2015)." This suggests that the weight set-point is not static and changes as nutrients become scarce or available (Muller et al, 2010).

> It is obvious that under Western lifestyle conditions, compensatory responses are passive rather than active and thus have a limited impact on body weight regulation (Meller, 2010).

A study done in 2011, called "Set-point Theory and Obesity" took a look at how people lowered their weight "set-point" through calorie restriction and weight loss surgery. The authors believed that gastric bypass surgery establishes a new weight set-point by altering caloric intake and feelings of fullness from the smaller stomach area (Farias, 2011). Weight regain after bariatric surgeries are common as patients slowly learn to over eat and stretch their stomachs. The weight set-point then reverts to its higher level and the patients gain weight.

The potato hack has numerous mechanisms by which it can effectively lower the weight set-point. A full belly with few calories may signal a dearth of available nutrients. At this point, the weight set-point would be lowered. In our early ancestry certain "fallback" foods were consumed when primary foods were not available (Marshall, 2007). For instance, in the African dry season, animals and fruits became scarce but underground yams were available. Though not a favored food, early hominids ate these starchy tubers to stave off starvation. It would not be an evolutionary advantage for resource-poor people to have ravaging hunger. Less hunger meant eating less so more would be available for others. While this seems like wild speculation on my part, I think I can show that the potato hack creates a condition in which starvation is sensed, but fat burning continues. In true starvation situations, the human body can limit the amount of fat burned as it attempts to conserve (McNamara, 1990).

Potatoes contain protease inhibitors (PI) considered by many to be "anti-nutrients (Novak, 2000)." Protease inhibitors are an evolutionary defense of plants to stop insect and herbivores from eating them. PIs are found in nearly all plants, so obviously the adaptation was not 100% effective. Potato protease inhibitors (PPI) are being studied for their ability to stimulate levels of cholecystokinin (CCK) in humans leading to increased levels of satiety. Cholecystokinin, as you may recall, is released from the intestinal lumen in response to ingestion of a meal. CCK has been shown to reduce food intake by stimulating satiety (Komarnytsky et al. 2011).

PPIs delay gastric emptying and slow the movement of food through the small intestine (Schwarz, 1994). This leads to a lessened effect on blood glucose and lingering feelings of fullness. Purified PPIs have been studied quite extensively as a review of the literature reveals. However, few studies have been performed using actual potato concentrates. Komarnytsky et al (2011) studied the effect of a PPI concentrate consisting of potato protease inhibitor II (PI2), potato protease inhibitor I, and potato kunitz-type protease inhibitor. These proteins are commonly found in all potatoes and have strong serine protease inhibitory activity.

> Metabolic syndrome and obesity are generally associated with an increased energy intake relative to calorie requirements and delayed satiation. Since changes in gastric motor and sensory functions in obesity may present useful targets to prevent and treat metabolic disorders, managing CCK-controlled gastric emptying and satiety could be a good strategy for reducing the risks associated with metabolic pathologies (Komarnytsky et al. 2011).

As you also may recall, CCK leads to gallbladder contractions (Yu, 1998). A danger of low fat diets is gallstones (Festi, 1998). As PPIs stimulate CCK and a reactive gallbladder emptying, this should not be a concern with the potato hack. Potato protease inhibitors (PPIs), not to be confused with proton pump inhibitors (PPIs), are a key factor in the weight set-point lower actions of the potato hack. Additionally, the "full-belly" signals and reduced calories are said to be behind much of the success of bariatric/gastric bypass surgery. This effect can readily be had from a short stint of the potato hack. Doctors are amazed when their bariatric patients are cured of T2 diabetes 24 hours after the surgery. You, too, will be amazed at the speed in which the potato hack exerts its effects!

References:

De Andrade, P. B., Neff, L. A., Strosova, M. K., Arsenijevic, D., Patthey-Vuadens, O., Scapozza, L., ... & Dorchies, O. M. (2015). Caloric restriction ...catch-up fat upon refeeding. *Frontiers in physiology*, *6*.

Farias, M. M., Cuevas, A. M., & Rodriguez, F. (2011). Set-point theory and obesity. *Metabolic syndrome and related disorders*, *9*(2), 85-89.

Festi, D., Colecchia, A., Orsini, M., Sangermano, A., Sottili, S., Simoni, P., ... & Petroni, M. L. (1998). Gallbladder motility and gallstone formation in obese patients following very low calorie diets. Use it (fat) to lose it (well). *International journal of obesity*, *22*(6), 592-600.

Harris, R. B. (1990). Role of set-point theory in regulation of body weight. *The FASEB Journal, 4*(15), 3310-3318.

Komarnytsky, S., Cook, A., & Raskin, I. (2011). Potato protease inhibitors inhibit food intake and increase circulating cholecystokinin levels by a trypsin-dependent mechanism. *International Journal of Obesity, 35*(2), 236-243.

Marshall, A. J., & Wrangham, R. W. (2007). Evolutionary consequences of fallback foods. *International Journal of Primatology, 28*(6), 1219-1235.

McNamara, J. M., & Houston, A. I. (1990). The value of fat reserves and the tradeoff between starvation and predation. *Acta biotheoretica, 38*(1), 37-61.

Müller, M. J., Bosy-Westphal, A., & Heymsfield, S. B. (2010). Is there evidence for a set point that regulates human body weight?. *F1000 medicine reports, 2*.

Novak, W. K., & Haslberger, A. G. (2000). Substantial equivalence of antinutrients and inherent plant toxins in genetically modified novel foods. *Food and Chemical Toxicology, 38*(6), 473-483.

Schwartz, J. G., Guan, D., Green, G. M., & Phillips, W. T. (1994). Treatment with an oral proteinase inhibitor slows gastric emptying and acutely reduces glucose and insulin levels after a liquid meal in type II diabetic patients. *Diabetes Care, 17*(4), 255-262.

Yu, P., Chen, Q., Xiao, Z., Harnett, K., Biancani, P., & Behar, J. (1998). Signal transduction pathways mediating CCK-induced gallbladder muscle contraction. *American Journal of Physiology-Gastrointestinal and Liver Physiology, 275*(2), G203-G211.

Extreme Low-fat Diet

It seems to make perfect sense. When you are fat you have extra body fat, so if you don't eat any dietary fat you will burn your body fat. The trouble is, life is seldom so simple. If losing weight was as simple as avoiding dietary fat, we'd all be thin.

Dietary fat is hard to avoid and is twice as calorie dense as protein and carbohydrate. The small amount of oil in an almond, for instance, overshadows the carbohydrate and protein. A handful of almonds a day will add about 15 grams of fat to your diet. The recommended daily allowance of fat, as advised by the Food and Nutrition Board of the National Institutes of Health is 25-35 grams per day. That handful of almonds represents *half* of your daily fat allowance.

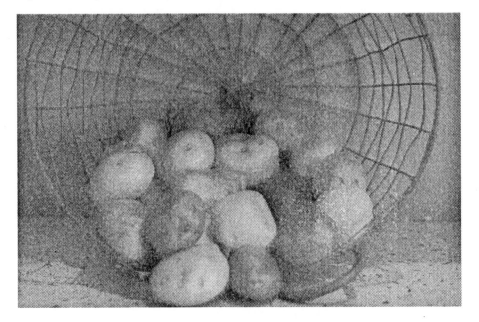

What we see recommended widely is a "low-fat" diet, but nowhere does anyone really ever define "low." Mainstream advice is to "choose low-fat foods," such as low-fat milk, "light" snacks, and fat-free dairy items. Eating in this fashion nearly guarantees you will end up eating more than the 25-35 grams recommended. 30 grams of fat has 270 calories (kcal). In a 2500 calorie per day diet, this represents just over 10% of calories from fat. For people eating the standard US diet filled with processed foods and snacks, it is very rare for anyone to eat just 10% of calories from fat. More likely, people eat 30% or more of their calories from fat. The average daily intake of fat is 33% for men and 32% for women based on 2009-2012 statistics collected by the Centers for Disease Control. Based on a 2500 kcal/day diet, this is over 92 grams of fat per day.

After decades of advice to eat low-fat choices, no real benefits have been seen on a population-wide basis, in fact, quite possibly our collective health is worse after this advice first became the norm in the 1970s. Low-fat foods such as margarine and snacks labeled "low-fat" have had deleterious effects on our health (Wansink and Chandon, 2006).

Kempner Rice Diet

Despite these glaring inconsistencies, there is also a body of research that suggests extremely low fat diets can be therapeutic in cases of metabolic derangement. The Kempner Rice Diet championed by Dr. Kempner in 1948 used a nearly zero fat diet to treat patients with hypertensive vascular disease. His diet used rice, sugar, and fruit and provided 2000 kcal per day with only 5 grams of fat (Kempner, 1948). Not only did Kempner's Rice Diet show dramatic reversals in hypertensive disease but also diabetes (Van Eck, 1959), cholesterol (Keys, 1950), and obesity (Chapman et al., 1950). Duke University used the Kempner Rice Diet successfully to remove excess fat from obese patients and also reported improvements in many metabolic markers (Newmark and Williamson, 1983).

Interest in the Kempner Rice Diet seems to have petered out in the 1950s. Despite the great results, even Kempner himself admitted the diet was nearly impossible for his patients to follow. Many have speculated that the efficacy of the rice diet in reducing hypertension was simply due to the reduction in dietary sodium, but perhaps the biggest failure of the Kempner Rice Diet was Kempner himself.

> I have whipped people in order to help them and because they say they want to be whipped (Kempner, 1997).

An article in the October 26, 1997 Spartanburg Herald-Journal gives an inside look at Kempner's depraved personality. He was sued in 1993 for the sexual harassment of a female employee who he whipped repeatedly with a riding crop and "used as a sex slave (Associated Press, 1997)." Had the "rice diet" had a better spokesman, it may have achieved more notice.

References:

Associated Press. (1997). Lawsuit reveals private life of rice diet doctor. Spartanburg Herald-Journal, October 26, 1997.

Chapman, C. B., Gibbons, T., & Henschel, A. (1950). The effect of the rice-fruit diet on the composition of the body. *New England Journal of Medicine, 243*(23), 899-905.

Kempner, W. (1948). Treatment of hypertensive vascular disease with rice diet. *The American journal of medicine, 4*(4), 545-577.

Keys, A., Mickelsen, O., Miller, E. V. O., & Chapman, C. B. (1950). The relation in man between cholesterol levels in the diet and in the blood. *American Association for the Advancement of Science. Science, 112*, 79-81.

Newmark, S. R., & Williamson, B. (1983). Survey of very-low-calorie weight reduction diets: I. Novelty diets. *Archives of internal medicine, 143*(6), 1195-1198.

Van Eck, W. F. (1959). The effect of a low fat diet on the serum lipids in diabetes and its significance in diabetic retinopathy. *The American journal of medicine, 27*(2), 196-211.

Wansink, B., & Chandon, P. (2006). Can "low-fat" nutrition labels lead to obesity?. *Journal of marketing research, 43*(4), 605-617.

Willett, W. C., Sacks, F., Trichopoulou, A., Drescher, G., Ferro-Luzzi, A., Helsing, E., & Trichopoulos, D. (1995). Mediterranean diet pyramid: a cultural model for healthy eating. *The American journal of clinical nutrition, 61*(6), 1402S-1406S.

1903 Irish Potato Diet for Diabetes Mellitus

A medical journal from 1903 describes feeding diabetic patients with large amounts of potatoes to alleviate symptoms of diabetes. Dr. Mosse noted that when he fed patients with large amounts (up to 6 pounds) of potatoes a day, their blood sugars normalized, thirst disappeared, and strength increased. Dr. Mosse surmised the large amounts of potash in potatoes may have been a key reason this plan worked (Ireland Royal Academy of Medicine (2013).

> Potatoes are generally held to be injurious in diabetes, and are usually placed in the list of forbidden articles. They are not only permissible, but even useful (Mosse, 1903).

Mosse's words from 1903 are still heard today. Advisors from all corners recommend avoidance of potatoes for those stricken with diabetes. Patients with well-controlled Type 1 and Type 2 diabetes as well as prediabetes are all cautioned to limit potato intake (Feinman et al., 2015). But is this the best advice?

Low-fat diets are all the rage, but very few are actually low in total fat intake. When we consciously avoid nearly all dietary fat for a short period of time, we quickly see increases in health markers and decreases in pro-inflammatory conditions. The potato hack is perfectly suited to inducing these positive changes. At the least, no one can say that a short term extreme low fat diet promotes inflammation or markers of poor health.

References:

Feinman, R. D., Pogozelski, W. K., Astrup, A., Bernstein, R. K., Fine, E. J., Westman, E. C., ... & Nielsen, J. V. (2015). Dietary carbohydrate restriction as the first approach in diabetes management: Critical review and evidence base. *Nutrition, 31*(1), 1-13.

Ireland Royal Academy Of Medicine. (2013). pp. 43-4. *Irish Journal of Medical Science, 1903* (Vol. 1). London: Forgotten Books. (Original work published 1903).

Calories in, Calories out

Calories in, Calories Out, or CICO, has been a proposed mechanism of weight loss since dieting first became popular in the 1700s. The father of modern dieting is probably the Rev. Sylvester Graham (1795-1851). You are undoubtedly familiar with his weight loss tool of choice, the Graham cracker. When Graham noted his parishioners getting fat eating the newly invented white bread, he formulated a cracker made of unsifted flour and advocated a vegetarian diet. Graham and his followers promoted the idea that to lose weight you simply eat less and move more.

The eat less, move more campaign is still going to this day, though it hardly helps many lose weight. Eating less and moving more are too subjective to be of much help, but the concepts are valid. With the potato hack, "moving more" is discouraged and weight loss is quite rapid.

At some point, an inquisitive scientist noted that there were 3500 calories (kcal) in one pound of pure dietary fat. This led to the faulty conclusion that eliminating 3500 kcal of total food intake would result in a fat loss of exactly one pound. This "3500 calorie rule" has infiltrated the healthcare and dieting industries and led to a nation of calorie counters.

The 3500 calorie rule is flawed on many levels. It does not take into account time or energy expenditure. A much better model of predictive weight loss uses a gradual caloric decrease over time:

> Every permanent 10-kcal change in energy intake/d will lead to an eventual weight change of 1 lb when the body weight reaches a new steady state (~100 kJ/d per kg of weight change). It will take nearly 1 y to achieve 50% and ~3 y to achieve 95% of this weight loss (Hall et al., 2011).

The potato hack is a calorie-restricted intervention. People will typically eat ½ of their normal calories or less per day. This often means a calorie deficit of 1000-2000 calories per day. Using the 3500 calorie rule, we would estimate a daily loss of approximately 1/3 − ½ pound. The actual values are closer to ½ − 1 pound per day. While the 3500 calorie rule is inherently flawed, a reduction in food intake should lead to a loss of body fat as the body burns stored fat for energy. When potato hacking, counting calories is much more precise. On the typical Western diet, an accurate calorie count is impossible (Malhotra et al., 2015). Serving sizes, perceived weights, and process differences lead to miscounting of calories

(Van Rijn, 2015).

During a potato hack, both CICO and the 3500 calorie rule can be used as the mechanism of weight loss, inaccurate as they are. During the normal diet, one may easily underestimate their daily intake, but when potato hacking, an accurate calorie count is very easy to achieve.

References:

Hall, K. D., Sacks, G., Chandramohan, D., Chow, C. C., Wang, Y. C., Gortmaker, S. L., & Swinburn, B. A. (2011). Quantification of the effect of energy imbalance on bodyweight. *The Lancet*, *378*(9793), 826-837.

Malhotra, A., DiNicolantonio, J. J., & Capewell, S. (2015). It is time to stop counting calories, and time instead to promote dietary changes that substantially and rapidly reduce cardiovascular morbidity and mortality. *Open heart*, *2*(1), e000273.

van Rijn, I., de Graaf, C., & Smeets, P. A. (2015). Tasting calories differentially affects brain activation during hunger and satiety. *Behavioural brain research*, *279*, 139-147.

Insulin Sensitivity

Many dieters are battling insulin resistance. When resistant to the effects of insulin, hunger, fat storage, and satiety are all impacted. Low carb diets are promoted as a way to avoid insulin spikes, but low carb diets can lead to a condition known as physiological insulin resistance (Ludwig, 2002). Insulin resistance is responsible for (Reaven, 1998):

- Brain fogginess and inability to focus.
- High blood sugar.
- Intestinal bloating — most intestinal gas is produced from carbohydrates in the diet, mostly those that humans cannot digest and absorb.
- Sleepiness, especially after meals.
- Weight gain, fat storage, difficulty losing weight — for most people, excess weight is from high fat storage; the fat in insulin resistant people is generally stored in and around abdominal organs in both males and females. It is currently suspected that hormones produced in that fat are a precipitating cause of insulin resistance.

- Increased blood triglyceride levels.
- Increased blood pressure. Many people with hypertension are either diabetic or pre-diabetic and have elevated insulin levels due to insulin resistance. One of insulin's effects is to control arterial wall tension throughout the body.
- Increased pro-inflammatory cytokines associated with cardiovascular disease.
- Depression. Due to the deranged metabolism resulting from insulin resistance, psychological effects, including depression, are not uncommon.
- Skin problems.

The conventional approach to treating insulin resistance is exercise and weight loss. When these fail to work, a low carb diet is often used in conjunction with drugs such as metformin and thiazolidinediones. Insulin resistance is often synonymous with pre-diabetes, but can rapidly progress to Type 2 Diabetes.

So how can a 3-5 days of the potato hack restore insulin sensitivity when it seems to require strict lifestyle changes and medical intervention? One explanation is that the gut microbiota play a significant role in obesity related inflammation and insulin resistance (Diamant, 2011). The potato hack has immediate and profound effects on inflammation. My own observations are that while on the potato hack, my FBG and postprandial glucose levels are much lower than normal.

Dietary interventions with resistant starch (RS), quickly restore balance and improve insulin sensitivity (Robertson, 2003). The potato hack is very high in RS. Insulin sensitivity is restored when the human body is forced to deal with carbohydrates in a controlled fashion. A continual flooding of sugars and starches is a quick route to insulin resistance and diabetes. A controlled feeding of potato followed by several hours of satiety-induced fasting allows the body to quickly shuffle all the carbohydrates into their proper place and begin to use body fat as a fuel source when the carbs are used up. This is exactly how we *are* designed to operate and exactly how we *do* operate on an all-potato hack.

The potato hack is also very good at eliminating body fat, in particular adipose fat. A recent study suggests that insulin sensitivity is impaired when the pancreas begins storing fat. As little as 1 gram of fat lost from the pancreas will restore insulin sensitivity (Lim, 2011). In this regard, the potato hack is also a very good intervention for reversing fatty liver disease and unsightly belly fat.

I am amazed at how quickly insulin sensitivity can be restored even in Type 2 Diabetic (T2D) patients. T2D can be reversed literally overnight following gastric bypass surgery. Many millions of people struggle needlessly while following their doctor's advice to avoid carbohydrates or medicate. Most of those with pre-diabetes will become T2D in a short while and most of those with T2D are never cured. The potato hack was once a valid treatment for diabetes in the days before medication was available.

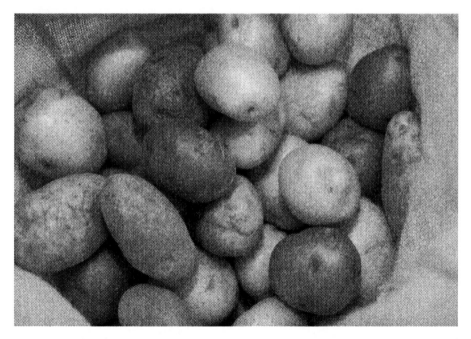

References:

Diamant, M., Blaak, E. E., & De Vos, W. M. (2011). Do nutrient–gut–microbiota interactions play a role in human obesity, insulin resistance and type 2 diabetes?. *Obesity Reviews, 12*(4), 272-281.

Lim, E. L., Hollingsworth, K. G., Aribisala, B. S., Chen, M. J., Mathers, J. C., & Taylor, R. (2011). Reversal of type 2 diabetes: normalisation of beta cell function in association with decreased pancreas and liver triacylglycerol. *Diabetologia, 54*(10), 2506-2514.

Ludwig, D. S. (2002). The glycemic index: physiological mechanisms relating to obesity, diabetes, and cardiovascular disease. *JAMA*, *287*(18), 2414-2423.

Reaven, G. M. (1988). Role of insulin resistance in human disease. *Diabetes*, *37*(12), 1595-1607.

Robertson, M. D., Currie, J. M., Morgan, L. M., Jewell, D. P., & Frayn, K. N. (2003). Prior short-term consumption of resistant starch enhances postprandial insulin sensitivity in healthy subjects. *Diabetologia*, *46*(5), 659-665.

Intestinal Microbiome

It has been well-established that resistant starch (RS) plays a huge part in health and weight loss. A large portion of the trillions of gut bugs that inhabit our large intestine prefer RS to any other food source and provide butyrate in return. Butyrate is a type of fat that can be used by the body itself to feed the cells which line the intestines, called colonocytes. When these cells are healthy, an environment is created in which hunger, weight, and overall health improves.

It is estimated that we need approximately 20-40 grams per day of resistant starch to produce enough butyrate to feel its effects on hunger and health (Ashwar, 2015, Topping, 2001). Most people rarely get over 5 grams of RS per day on a typical diet (Nugent, 2005). A large cooked potato that weighs ½ pound, has approximately 2 grams of RS—hardly enough to keep our gut bugs occupied. However, 3 pounds of cooked and cooled potatoes, reheated or eaten cold, contain a whopping 60 grams of RS! Three pounds of potato, if all eaten freshly cooked, still have about 12 grams of RS, three times the average intake of most people in the world. Anyone who tries the potato hack is undoubtedly, for the first time in their life, experiencing what it feels like to have received a meaningful dose of RS.

The paper, "Butyrate and Propionate Protect against Diet-Induced Obesity and Regulate Gut Hormones via Free Fatty Acid Receptor 3-Independent Mechanisms," describes the mechanisms behind a huge burst of short chain fatty acids (such as butyrate and propionate) as seen in the potato hack, this study concludes (Lin, 2012):

In summary, the present findings demonstrate butyrate and propionate regulate gut hormone release, suppress food intake, and protect against diet-induced obesity. We also show that FFAR3 is required for maximal GLP-1 induction by butyrate, but is dispensable for butyrate – and propionate-dependent effects on body weight and GIP stimulation. As enteroendocrine nutrient-sensing and the incretin axis are subjects of intense interest in drug discovery for metabolic disorders, future studies to determine the signaling mechanisms responsible for SCFAs' beneficial effects may have a major impact on the development of novel therapies for diabetes and obesity.

Another pertinent paper, "Regulation of inflammation by short chain fatty acids," explains the relationship between short-chain fatty acids produced by gut bacteria concludes (Vinolo, 2011): "Therapeutic application of these fatty acids for the treatment of inflammatory pathologies is also highlighted."

I go more in depth into the intestinal microbiome in the resistant starch chapter, but I am convinced that possibly the greatest impact of the potato hack is from RS. Resistant starch holds great promise for getting the world out of the mess it's in with regards to poor gut health. The potato hack is the only dietary intervention in the world that supplies such a massive dose of RS.

References:

Ashwar, B. A., Gani, A., Shah, A., Wani, I. A., & Masoodi, F. A. (2015). Preparation, health benefits and applications of resistant starch—A review. *Starch-Stärke*

Lin, H. V., Frassetto, A., Kowalik Jr, E. J., Nawrocki, A. R., Lu, M. M., Kosinski, J. R., ... & Marsh, D. J. (2012). Butyrate and propionate protect against diet-induced obesity and regulate gut hormones via free fatty acid receptor 3-independent mechanisms. *PLoS One, 7*(4), e35240.

Nugent, A. P. (2005). Health properties of resistant starch. *Nutrition Bulletin, 30*(1), 27-54.

Topping, D. L., & Clifton, P. M. (2001). Short-chain fatty acids and human colonic function: roles of resistant starch and nonstarch polysaccharides. *Physiological reviews, 81*(3), 1031-1064.

Vinolo, M. A., Rodrigues, H. G., Nachbar, R. T., & Curi, R. (2011). Regulation of inflammation by short chain fatty acids. *Nutrients*, *3*(10), 858-876.

Food Reward Theories

Human brains have developed "reward centers" which were very important to early man who needed every calorie he could get, but these same chemical reactions that helped us survive famines and ice ages are now making us fat. Many new diets are based on studies of sensory-specific satiety, or the tendency to feel full and stop eating when flavors are limited.

Research shows that different types of flavors, such as sweet, salty, and sour, activate their own appetite centers in the brain, which is why you might feel full after eating a savory meal but still have room for dessert. One popular theory is that once you turn on an appetite center, you must eat until it registers fullness. If you turn on many centers at once, you must eat until they're all full (Singh, 2014).

Other food reward theories suggest that hyper-palatable foods override our sense of being hungry. There is a "motivational component" tied to the mesolimbic dopamine system, the same system that leads people to obsessive sex, gambling, and substance abuse (Appelhans, 2011). The potato hack takes away all distractions of these hyper-palatable foods. Many people have reported that for the first time they can remember, while doing the potato hack, they are simply not hungry.

For binge eaters, or anyone who can't say "no" to a request for supersizing the fries, the potato hack can be a welcome respite in a world where we are constantly bombarded with tasty food treats. Food manufacturers know that most humans cannot resist the allure of appealing food. Take back control with the potato hack.

References:

Appelhans, B. M., Woolf, K., Pagoto, S. L., Schneider, K. L., Whited, M. C., & Liebman, R. (2011). Inhibiting food reward: delay discounting, food reward sensitivity, and palatable food intake in overweight and obese women. *Obesity*, *19*(11), 2175-2182.

Singh, M. (2014). Mood, food, and obesity. *Frontiers in psychology*, *5*.

POTATO QUOTES

"THE PASTY TASTE, THE NATURAL INSIPIDITY, THE UNHEALTHY QUALITY OF (THE POTATO), WHICH IS FLATULENT AND INDIGESTIBLE, HAS CAUSED IT TO BE REJECTED FROM REFINED HOUSEHOLDS AND RETURNED TO THE PEOPLE, WHOSE COARSE PALATES AND STRONGER STOMACHS ARE SATISFIED WITH ANYTHING CAPABLE OF APPEASING HUNGER."

LEGRAND D'AUSSY (1783)

FROM 'CONSUMING PASSIONS', JONATHON GREEN EDITOR (1985)

Notes:

PART 3

RESISTANT STARCH AND GUT HEALTH

CHAPTER 9. THE MAGIC OF RESISTANT STARCH

Resistant starch (RS) should be a "hack" of its own. I figured at the very least, it deserved a chapter of its own. Shortly after learning that potatoes could induce rapid weight loss, I found that they contain very high levels of RS. It's quite likely that the entire success of the potato hack is due to the high RS content of potatoes.

Potatoes contain two types of starch: amylose and amylopectin. These starches are generally found in a 20:80 ratio favoring amylopectin. Potato starch is granulated in such a way that digestive enzymes cannot degrade the starch molecules. Therefore, we can say:

> Resistant starch (RS) is starch that does not get digested in the stomach or small intestine and enters the large intestine intact.

This bland definition may be one of the most important things you ever read. This seemingly innocuous substance known as "resistant starch" is a simple solution to a huge problem—the feeding of our intestinal microbiome. For decades now, resistant starch has been exhaustively studied and declared time and again an ideal solution to many of modern society's health woes. If you find yourself saying, "Why am I just now hearing about this?" you are not alone.

The next question I hope you'll ask is, "Do I really need resistant starch?" The answer is, "Most likely!"

You may recognize yourself as having the modern, dyspeptic gut I've repeatedly described: Frequent heartburn, loose stools or constipation, indigestion, smelly gas, Gastroesophageal Reflux Disease (GERD), Irritable Bowel Syndrome (IBS), or worse. You may even have one of the many autoimmune diseases that are running rampant, diabetes, metabolic syndrome, or cancer.

Digestive diseases affect over 70 million people in the US alone! These diseases required 48.3 million ambulatory care visits, 21.7 million hospitalizations, and caused 245,921 deaths in 2009. Total costs for digestive diseases is estimated at $300 billion. These stats are getting worse, not better.

It's estimated that over 90 million Americans use antacids or other digestive upset medicines. Upset stomachs are the number one cause of self-treatment, and those late-night trips to Walmart yield an impressive display of over-the-counter offerings for the modern, dyspeptic human gut.

If none of these describe you, then you have somehow discovered a way to feed your gut flora and you have managed to collect a diverse supply of happy gut microbes—good job! But, if you aren't happy with your gastrointestinal tract or immunity, increasing resistant starch in your diet may be just the ticket. There is so much known about resistant starch by food scientists, yet it is an unknown entity to the people that could benefit from it.

The Revolution that Never Was

> One of the major developments in our understanding of the importance of carbohydrates for health in the past twenty years has been the discovery of resistant starch.
>
> — Joint Food and Agricultural Organization of the United Nations/World Health Organization, 1997

The definition normally used for RS is nearly the exact same definition that is used for "dietary fiber," and a huge reason that RS has escaped the attention of the medical community and the public. Resistant starch is not your normal dietary fiber, although it shares similar properties. RS could more technically be called "fermentable starch" or "prebiotic starch," but since its discovery in 1982, it has been called "resistant starch." The health implications of RS were not immediately seen, and it's only been in the last 5-10 years that the huge impact RS can make on the health of humans has been explored. The pioneers in RS as a health booster were pig farmers looking for a way to raise antibiotic-free pigs. They found that pigs fed raw potatoes had less infections than pigs fed standard foods. Were it not for this attention, RS may have gone unnoticed to this day.

Resistant starch differs from fiber in many ways and should not be confused with the dietary fiber listed on nutrition labels. Let's look at a standard definition for dietary fiber.

Dietary fiber is the indigestible portion of food derived from plants. There are two main components:

- Soluble fiber dissolves in water. It is readily fermented in the colon into gases and physiologically active byproducts, and can be prebiotic and/or viscous. Soluble fibers tend to slow the movement of food through the system.

- Insoluble fiber does not dissolve in water. It can be metabolically inert and provide either stool bulking or metabolically ferment (probiotic action) in the large intestine. Bulking fibers absorb water as they move through the digestive system, easing defecation. Fermentable insoluble fibers mildly promote stool regularity, although not to the extent that bulking fibers do, but they can be readily fermented in the colon into gases and physiologically active byproducts. Insoluble fibers tend to accelerate the movement of food through the system.

By this definition, RS seems to be just another type of dietary fiber—but to call it that, and lump it together with all other dietary fibers was one of the biggest blunders of all time. I hope that the attention RS is getting these days spurs people into action for getting RS classified as an important food ingredient that deserves its own special place on nutrition labels and in people's minds.

In 2003, the World Health Organization attempted to define the perfect diet for world-wide health in their publication, *Population nutrient intake goals for preventing diet-related chronic diseases*. They made numerous recommendations on dietary fat, sugars, carbohydrates and protein, but when it came to fiber, they admitted defeat in light of new information concerning RS:

> The best definition of dietary fibre remains to be established, given the potential health benefits of resistant starch.

This statement, made over 13 years ago, has massive implications for world health and displays the incredible ignorance of modern medicine. At this behest, RS should have become a household word during the last decade. Let's not wait another decade for the next sound-bite, let's do something about it NOW.

Five Types of Resistant Starch

Resistant starch has been classified into five general types named RS1–RS5, described below:

Type 1 –

RS1 is the physically inaccessible starch that is locked within cell walls such as the shells of nuts, seed coatings and hulls, and other food matrixes. Milling and chewing can make these starches more accessible and less resistant. While eating whole seeds is very healthy for our digestive systems, RS1 is not an important food source for gut microbes since many of these protective structures cannot be breached and they pass through the body completely undigested. When the coating is breached, RS1 becomes RS2.

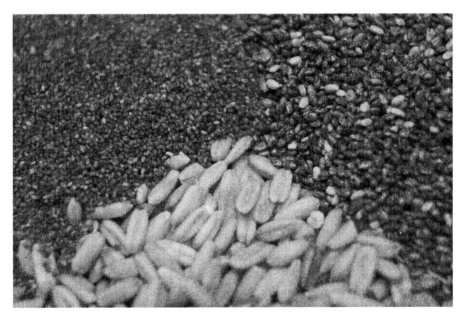

RS Type 1 – Chia Seeds, Teff, Oats (Author's Photo)

Type 2 –

RS2 is in raw starch granules, sometimes called "native starch." These starch granules are protected from digestion by the structure and composition of the starch granule itself. The structure of the starch granules has an impact on the resistance of the starch—such as the shape of the granule, size of pores or susceptibility of the starch to germinate. Their compact structure prevents digestive enzymes and stomach acid from attacking the starch allowing it to reach the large intestine whole. When RS2 is heated above a certain point, usually around 140 degrees F, it swells and bursts losing its RS value completely. RS2 is found in potatoes, green bananas, plantains, taro, cassava, and in most cereal grains. Not all raw starch is resistant starch. Corn and rice starch, for instance are readily digestible for the most part. Potatoes and plantains contain the most resistant starches in nature although there are other good candidates such as mung bean starch and lotus seed starch.

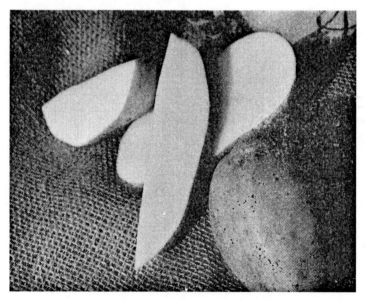

RS Type 2 – Raw Potatoes (Author's Photo)

Type 3 –

RS3 is retrograded or crystallized starch formed after cooking. This is the starch found in cooked and cooled potatoes, bread crusts, cornflakes, and cold sushi rice. RS3 is non-granular starch that resists digestion. RS3 is interesting because it can withstand heat once it has formed. In most cooking methods, RS2 is destroyed and RS3 takes its place, becoming more dense after repeated heating and cooling cycles. RS3 is the most interesting type of RS and this property to 'retrograde' is easily exploited. When fully retrograded, the starch forms a double helix, much like our DNA, and binds water in the interior spaces of the structure. After a few hours in storage, the helices undergo an aggregation and form gels which are thermally stable and resistant to attack by digestive enzymes. In the colon, RS3 acts like slowly digestible/low glycemic starches do in the small intestine—burns long and slow, spreading its influence to the distal ends of the colon.

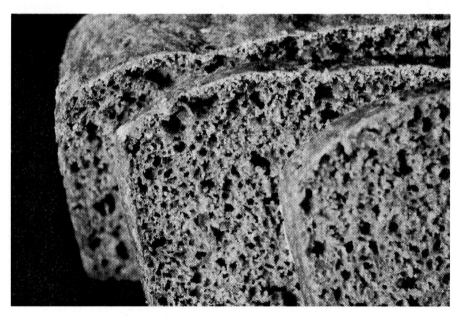

RS Type 3 – Tim's Homemade Whole Grain Bread (Author's Photo)

Type 4/5 –

RS4 and 5 are man-made, chemically modified or re-polymerized starch. It is not found in nature, but rather manufactured and used widely in the food industry to alter the characteristics of starch to decrease its digestibility. RS4 can be produced by chemical modifications, such as conversion, substitution, or cross-linking, which can prevent its digestion by blocking enzyme access and forming atypical linkages. RS4 does seem to exhibit the same properties as natural RS2 and RS3, so it shouldn't be dismissed entirely because it is man-made. RS5 is made by heating and cooling starches in the presence of fat. Re-heating cooled rice or potatoes in oil is an easy at-home method of RS5 creation. This type(s) of RS is used widely by the food industry to give processed foods an engineered taste or to extend shelf-life. Until the science is clear, I'd suggest staying away from RS4 and 5 and focusing on RS1, 2, and 3 from real food.

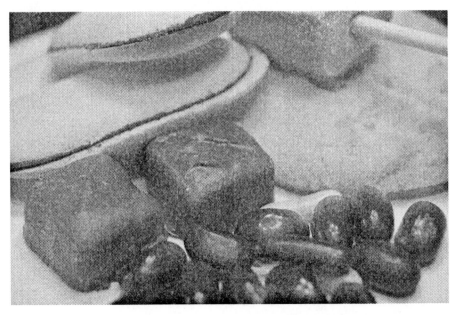

RS Types 4/5 – Jackie's Candy Stash (Author's Photo)

Which RS Type is Best?

RS1 is a bit awkward since it's only as resistant as it's outer shell. Once the shell is breached, it becomes RS2 and then RS3 if cooked. RS4 is also a bit strange; it's a man-made substance and readily used by the food manufacturing industry to add texture and extend shelf life of prepared foods while allowing them to list the food item as "high in fiber." No one should look to RS4 to fill their need for resistant starch, our ancestors certainly didn't!

Eating whole seeds as found in berries or flaxseed can deliver a nice dose of RS to your colon, but not everyone has the bacteria required to break down the hard outer shell of seeds. If seeds are a common part of your diet, eventually you will be able to utilize the RS1 found inside seeds as you develop the bacteria needed to "crack" these seeds open. Most people find grinding seeds makes them much more digestible, but you cut the RS in half.

RS2 and RS3 are the prehistoric powerhouses that fueled our gut microbes for millions of years. As you can imagine, when we were living a very primitive life we ate our starches raw, consuming only RS2, then later as we learned to cook, RS3 was introduced to the mix. For at least a million years, we likely ate a combination of RS2 and RS3 with hunger and glee. After routine use of controlled fire and larger human settlements, RS3 was undoubtedly used to wean babies, provide consistent meals and energy, and to feed busy hunters and pastoralists. You can bet that at the ancestral hearth, leftovers were not scorned!

Scientific studies show there are slight but significantly noted differences in the two types of RS:

- RS3 was shown to dilute fecal ammonia and other fecal carcinogens whereas RS2 does not unless combined with significant amounts of insoluble fiber to bulk stools.

- RS3 was shown to increase absorption of magnesium, calcium and phosphorous in pigs compared to RS2 (but lowered it in rats).

- RS2 and RS3 have mixed results in initiation and promotion stage in colon carcinogenesis and human colorectal cancer trials however stale cooked maize porridge (RS3) consumed by native Africans was highly associated with protection against colorectal cancer.

- RS3 and starch intakes [but not conventional fiber (NSP)] in epidemiological observations demonstrate 25-50% relative risk reductions in colorectal neoplasms and cancer incidence.

- RS3 was better than RS2 or RS4 at relieving symptoms of constipation.

- RS3 shifts nitrogen excretion from urine to feces better than RS2, implying that RS3 is better for people with kidney or liver impairments than RS2.

- RS2 showed markedly better growth of Eubacterium rectale, a species associated with high butyrate production, when compared to RS4. Extraordinary increases bifidobacteria were associated with RS4 (10-fold in several human subjects).

Most of the hundreds of studies done over the past 30 years use RS2 from corn or potatoes as their source and see favorable results. RS3, when studied, was mostly in the form of retrograded corn or tapioca starch. Very few studies looked at the benefits of one RS source over another. I think it is prudent to include both RS2 and RS3 in your diet for the bulk of your RS needs, but don't shy away from RS1 as intact seeds, legumes and whole grains or gluten-free (GF) grains which have benefits of their own. A natural approach is probably best when it emulates your individual ancestral eating patterns...consume most of your starches fresh, cooked-cooled and some raw. Supplements can maintain or help meet health goals.

But, But, Isn't RS a Dreaded FODMAP???

Some of you don't know what a FODMAP is?

FODMAP is an acronym for "Fermentable, Oligo-, Di, and Mono-saccharides, And Polyols." This is a diet for people with bowel disorders, developed to limit FODMAPs. It is said to relieve symptoms for many; the trouble is, many of the FODMAPs are potent prebiotics and eliminating these compounds essentially starves the gut flora. While this may have short-term therapeutic benefits, it is not healthy in the long-run if gut health is your main concern.

Technically, RS is not a FODMAP, but the "F" kind of catches it as a fermentable substance. Really, it could have just as easily been called the "F" diet—not for the grade I give it, but for the avoidance of all things fermentable.

If you are following a strict no FODMAP diet, you'll want to add RS to the list. You'll also want to re-evaluate your reasons for avoiding all food for your gut bugs—it's cruel and unusual punishment for trillions of hapless bystanders. While you may enjoy the relief afforded by FOD-MAP restriction it is at great cost to your gut flora. Seek and destroy the offending pathogens and start eating prebiotics as soon as you can.

The Father of RS

Hans N. Englyst coined the term "resistant starch" in 1982 while attempting to measure dietary fiber. He found that certain starch granules hindered his attempts to recreate digestion in a test tube and labeled the undigested portions of starch "resistant starch." It seems at this point, RS was little more than a nuisance to researchers, but Englyst went on to publish dozens of papers discussing RS and ways to measure it.

At first, Englyst used ileostomy patients to measure RS. Ileostomy patients provide a perfect way to test for undigested starches because all of the food that leaves their small intestine is collected in a pouch and can be examined for anything that escaped digestion. Many of the RS content lists that were developed by Englyst using the ileostomy method are used to today as the "gold standard" to compared more modern methods of RS testing against.

How much RS is in this?

One reason you won't be seeing RS listed on nutrition labels any time soon is because it's so hard to measure. Take the potato for instance, the RS content changes drastically as the raw potato is cooked, cooled, and reheated numerous times. The variety of potato and cooking methods also impact the RS content. Except for the case of highly processed snack foods and bakery items, it's better to simply learn which foods are rich in RS and how to best prepare them to maximize RS for your health.

Several different methods have been developed to measure the RS content in foods beyond a simple examination of ileostomy bags:

- The Berry Method derived from Englyst' experiments using pancreatic enzymes from pigs proved unreliable.
- The Champ method modified the Berry method to correct for pH and temperature and gave consistent RS measurements.

- Muir and O'Dea used a similar method, but the food was first chewed by human volunteers.

- Bednar and associates developed a method in 2001 to measure RS using dogs with modified digestive systems and surgically implanted tubes to measure RS at different stages. This method was very accurate but not very popular.

- AOAC Method 2002.02 is now the standard method for measuring RS.

The Association of Official Agricultural Chemists adopted this method in 2002, and describe the method:

> Starch is solubilized and hydrolyzed to glucose by the combined action of pancreatic-amylase and amyloglucosidase (AMG) for 16 h at 37°C. The reaction is terminated by addition of ethanol or industrial methylated spirits (IMS) and RS is recovered as a pellet by centrifugation. RS in the pellet is dissolved in 2M KOH by vigorously stirring in an ice–water bath. This solution is neutralized with acetate buffer and the starch is quantitatively hydrolyzed to glucose with AMG. Glucose is measured with glucose oxidase–peroxidase reagent (GOPOD), which is a measure of RS content. Nonresistant starch (solubilized starch) is determined by pooling the original supernatant and the washings and measuring the glucose content with GOPOD.

Even with this agreed-upon measuring standard in effect, differences are seen between testing labs and the terminology used makes it all very confusing for the average consumer.

Prior to adopting this standard, the AOAC sent identical samples of green banana, potato starch, corn starch, corn flakes, kidney beans, and several types of RS4 to 37 different labs for independent testing. The results were fairly consistent, but quite variable. For instance, the raw potato starch showed an average RS content of 63% on a "% as is" basis, with the ranges being between 56% and 76%.

To add to the complication, all of the labs present their data in three ways: "As-is basis," "Dry-weight basis," and "RS as a percentage of total starch." When compared with these three terms, raw potato starch from 37 different labs is expressed like this:

RS Content of Raw Potato Starch, AOAC Method 2002.02

- As-is basis – 63%
- Dry-weight basis – 72%
- RS as a percentage of total starch – 73%
- For reference, here are the RS contents of raw potato starch using the various other testing procedures: (all expressed as a percentage of total starch)
- Ileostomy patient studies—up to 83%.
- The Champ method—87.5%.
- Models that use human volunteers to pre-chew food—66%.
- Canine models of digestion—68%.

As you can see, pinning down the actual value of RS is not an extremely accurate science. With the AOAC testing standard in place, we at least have a common reference for all RS tests.

Another issue with RS testing, especially for RS3, is that the test method calls for heating and cooling cycles which skew the results by forming more RS3 than was in the original sample.

What can RS do for me?

Hundreds of studies have been conducted over the last 30 years on the effects of RS to:

- Improve bowel health
- Lower pH
- Increase epitheleal thickness
- Kill cancer cells
- Lower postprandial glycemia
- Increase insulin sensitivity
- Reduce body weight and prevent weight regain
- Decrease inflammation in the intestines and entire body

- Reduce risk of breast cancer and colorectal cancer
- Reduce cholesterol/triglycerides
- Increase production of brain neurotransmitters serotonin and melatonin
- Remove certain pathogens from small intestine
- Preserve Vitamin D in the body
- Increase mineral and vitamin production and uptake
- Remove toxins and heavy metals from the bloodstream
- Increase satiety and regulate hunger hormones
- Reduce fat storage after meals
- Improve the gut microbiome (synergy, prebiotic, symbiotic)
- Protect probiotic bacteria

Looking closely at the list of studied benefits of RS, you can almost see a linear progression from its simple physical properties to its in-depth role in maintaining a healthy gut microbiome. This is also exactly how biological science has progressed during the same time as newer methods to test gut microbes come to light. Many of the older studies that yielded mixed results are being done again with a focus on how RS affects the microbiome and when looked at in that way, the studies prove successful or shed light on why they failed.

Here are a few of the more common, well-studied, and much sought-after results of increasing RS in your diet:

Glucose Response and Insulin Sensitivity:

Probably the most widely studied effect of RS and one of its biggest "selling points" is in its control of blood sugar. From a well-documented "second-meal effect" to complete reversal of Type 2 Diabetes, RS could be a godsend for many and is being studied extensively for ways to bring it to the masses. Studies looking at different types of RS, found that they are equally effective at controlling postprandial blood glucose spikes and that RS exerts a stability in blood glucose levels.

Other notable studies have shown increases in "whole body insulin sensitivity." Since insulin resistance is closely associated with complications of diabetes and heart disease this remains at the forefront of RS research. The blood sugar changes that are seen when RS is incorporated into the diet can be compared to the blood sugar changes seen when diabetics undergo gastric bypass surgery, an almost immediate increase in insulin sensitivity results and is closely associated with changes to the microbiome of intestinal bacteria.

Body Weight Regulation:

As a diet aid, RS will fall short. It's not as simple as taking a diet pill and the studies in this area have shown mixed results. What is very apparent in the studies of RS and weight is that a when gut bugs are fed RS, they will do everything in their power to help get you to a lean, healthy state. Studies that look simply at weight often fail to see reductions because RS can actually lead to a heavier, thicker, healthier intestinal tract and increase the numbers of bacteria living there—a weight gain everyone should be happy with. Another interesting field of research into RS has to do with re-gaining weight lost through exercise; it was found that after losing a considerable bit of fat, keeping it off was easier with RS than with continued exercise—and certainly intestinal microbe driven through better hunger signals and fat storage hormones. What is really exciting is that the addition of RS, post weight loss, clearly showed a trend toward muscle growth and away from fat storage—the main goals for improving insulin sensitivity.

You may have heard of "cortisol," a stress hormone that often stymies weight loss and muscle building progress. Well, cortisol is no match for RS...cortisol is lowered on an RS supplemented diet and helps explain the reduction in weight regain and also has been implicated in wholebody energy metabolism. The cortisol connection is entirely driven by gut bugs and is possibly one of their most important contributions to our overall health.

Inflammation:

There are several studies looking at the anti-inflammatory effects of RS, and almost every study on gut microbes addresses the fact that gut bacteria play a huge role in lowering inflammation. The studies in which inflammation were addressed showed conclusively that the addition of RS to the diet decreased inflammation in the intestines and body-wide. This area will undoubtedly be explored further as new evidence on the connection between gut bugs and inflammation come to light. Inflammation is characteristic of heart disease, diabetes, obesity, and many other diseases. RS is one of the keys to unlocking the mystery behind inflammation.

Cholesterol and Triglycerides:

Chronic RS intake reduces levels of LDL (bad) cholesterol and triglycerides. That's really all you need to know. But in case you love facts, RS also lowers fasting serum triglycerides and cholesterol levels and RS lowers levels of liver triglycerides and cholesterol as well as triglycerides found in adipose (fat) tissue. Furthermore, genes in the liver which control cholesterol production were lower and genes which clear cholesterol were higher after continued feedings of RS.

Bowel Health:

Early investigations into RS focused on positive changes to the colonic environment such as lowered pH and elevated production of butyrate. Both of these changes decrease levels of pathogenic intestinal microbes and improve bowel functions. As more research is done on the positive effects of a well-fed gut microbiome, the importance of RS has been elevated to epic proportions. Many of the old studies from the 80s and 90s are being re-created with a focus on gut bugs and through test methods for gut microbes that didn't exist back then. The studies are proving very insightful.

In numerous early studies, researchers were confused as to why the results of RS experiments varied widely between study participants. Modern studies looking at microbes eating RS have discovered that certain key microbes must be in place before RS can be fully utilized. For instance, when a gut microbe known as Ruminococcus bromii is thriving, RS causes massive increases in the beneficial gut microbes Bifidobacterium and Bacillus species. When Ruminococcus bromii is absent, no change in Bifidobacterium or Bacillus is detected. This discovery led to new theories on the fermentation of RS by gut bacteria. One theory, known as the "Keystone Species Theory" describes that RS is not fermented simply by many different microbes, but selectively targeted by only a few "keystone" species. The byproducts are then consumed by RS co-feeders in a remarkable progression of events which leads to the production of important chemicals and compounds important to intestinal health.

Cancer:

Nearly all of the studies done on RS in the last 3 years have been centered around cancer prevention and cures—and not just colorectal cancer, but also breast cancer and the use of RS as a chemotherapy enhancer.

RS has been shown to reduce the survival of human colon cancer cells through its stimulation of short-chain fatty acids. When cancer cells are exposed to high doses of RS boosted butyrate, they are killed through DNA fragmentation, also known as cell apoptosis. A diet high in RS has been shown to prevent the formation of cancer cells altogether.

A few years back, lots of press was given to the reports that red meat consumption causes cancer. What wasn't widely disseminated were the studies that showed when RS was fed alongside red meat, the cancers never formed and the damaging effects of meat were totally negated and that the intestinal cells that are at risk for meat-induced damage were made much healthier with the inclusion of RS.

Researchers often inject animals with powerful carcinogens and assess their health after testing anti-cancer protocols. One such study looked at the effects of raw starches (RS2) and man-made starches (RS4) comparing their anti-cancer properties. In a head-to-head comparison, the raw starches beat the man-made starches in fermentation and anti-cancer properties. However, in another study, both RS2 and RS4 were equally effective at providing cancer protection.

Due to its "resistant" nature, RS is being used in chemotherapy to protect cancer drugs from digestive processes and to target colon cancer cells. When drugs are coated with an RS layer of a particular thickness, a precise targeting method is produced with profound impact on the treatment of bowel cancer.

And lastly, breast cancer is seeing the benefits of RS therapy. Breast cancer is a huge concern for women on estrogen therapy—recent mouse studies have shown a decrease in breast cancer cells and improvements to how their bodies metabolized circulating estrogen. To get the benefits of RS for breast and other cancers, one simply has to eat RS rich foods.

Preserves Vitamin D:

Another very recent discovery is that when eating a diet high in RS, symptoms of vitamin D deficiency are ameliorated. This is especially important for Type 1 and Type 2 diabetics with impaired kidneys who excrete excess vitamin D in their urine. Diabetes is becoming an epidemic and RS has been shown to mitigate the effects of diabetes, and may eventually prove to be the cure.

Adherence/Encapsulation Technology:

An interesting advancement in RS technology has been its synergistic effects when combined with live probiotic bacteria prior to consumption. Resistant starch displays an amazing ability to "capture" nearby microbes through a process known as ligand mimicry. This same process that is used to treat cholera patients is also used to package probiotic microbes in the supplement industry.

Through a modern invention known as "microencapsulation," tiny beads of RS are coated with beneficial bacterial strains and they, in turn, are coated with more RS. This provides protection and food for the live organisms to survive lengthy storage times on the shelf and also provides protection from harsh stomach acid and digestive enzymes which normally destroy live bacteria destined for the large intestine. Early attempts at this synergistic feature of RS and probiotics were undertaken using ice cream with a high RS content to capitalize on the effects of low temperature on the survival of probiotic strains of microbes. However, these methods have been replaced in favor of microencapsulation, although the ice cream method has returned recently and a 2013 study showed it may prove highly stable.

For the adventurous home-enthusiast of RS consumption, the property of RS to preserve microbes can be used to increase the effectiveness of your expensive probiotic supplements. Simply mix your probiotics supplements with a cold liquid containing a tablespoonful of a raw starch such as potato, plantain, or tapioca starch, stir and drink. Probiotic pills in capsule form can be emptied into the mixture for good effect. If you are a consumer of yogurt, kefir, kombucha, or kvass, adding a spoonful of RS to the mix will increase the likelihood of the bacteria present in these getting to, and making a home in, your large intestine.

How much do we eat? What about everyone else?

As worldwide cancer and disease rates climb, researchers have been examining the diets of different populations. One thing modern civilizations have in common is their distinct lack of RS. In 2004, the AOAC conducted a survey and found the worldwide consumption of RS was 7 grams per day, with the United States and western European countries on the lower end and less developed countries at the higher end.

- Sweden – 3.2g
- United States – 4.9g
- Australia – 5.3g
- Italy – 8.5g
- China – 14.9g

Stale Maize Porridge

There are so many factors in play here that there can be no simple correlations. However, a really great study was done in 2007 to compare the relatively high rates of colorectal cancer among African Americans and the very low rates found in Native Africans living a simple, rural life.

In this study, the diets and lifestyles of 17 African American and 18 Native Africans were examined. The colorectal cancer rates between these groups was less than 1 in 10,000 for the Native Africans and 65 in 10,000 for the African Americans. During the intense scrutiny, several glaring disparities were evident: notably the Native Africans were consuming much more resistant starch. A staple in the Native African diet was cornmeal porridge which was their main source of carbohydrates and approximately 20% resistant starch. Their intake was close to 50 grams per day of RS compared to the African American intake of less than 5 grams per day.

An examination of the rural African diet showed that it was relatively lacking in dietary fiber but very high in RS which ensures their colons remain very resilient to cancer formation. Interestingly, it's not only the choice of food (maize porridge) but the traditional preparation method that makes it so high in RS. Typically, the maize porridge is made by heating cornmeal in boiling water. The finished product is then stored for days and consumed cold—this leads to the formation of retrograded

RS3. When consumed is fermented into the short-chain fatty acids such as butyrate and propionate leading to increased numbers of beneficial gut bacteria and healthier colons almost completely lacking in signs of inflammation and cancer.

Furthermore, these same groups of stale maize porridge eaters were studied in 1986 where it was determined that the simple, high fiber diet significantly lowered fecal pH, an indicator of gut health, and protected the connoisseur of such tasty fare from colorectal cancer.

The Australian Paradox

Earlier we said, "don't confuse resistant starch with dietary fiber." The Australian Paradox illustrates our point. Nearly 30 years ago, Australia was faced with a crisis—they had one of the highest rates of colorectal (bowel) cancer among all 'civilized' nations. When they examined what the average Australian was eating, it was clear that they lacked dietary fiber. The Australian Commonwealth Scientific and Industrial Research Organisation (CSIRO), the Australian federal government agency for scientific research, began a systematic approach to increasing the fiber intakes of Australians. Through research, advertising, and training Australians now eat more fiber per capita than any other Western nation... and they still have the highest rate of bowel cancer. Clearly something is wrong! This seeming mismatch has been termed, "The Australian Paradox." A high fiber diet should lead to reduced risk of colorectal cancer, not increased.

Rural Native Africans eating a very basic diet high in resistant starch and low in dietary fiber have a colorectal cancer rate of less than 1 in 10,000. Australians eating a diet low in RS and high in dietary fiber have a colorectal cancer rate of 1 in 12.

As you can imagine, CSIRO is shifting their focus from dietary fiber to resistant starch. They have issued a recommendation of 20 grams of RS per day, the first such recommendation in the world, and have begun partnerships with food producers to increase RS in the food supply. While RS may not be the ultimate solution to the Australian Paradox, emulating a diet where colorectal cancer is nearly unheard of is a good start.

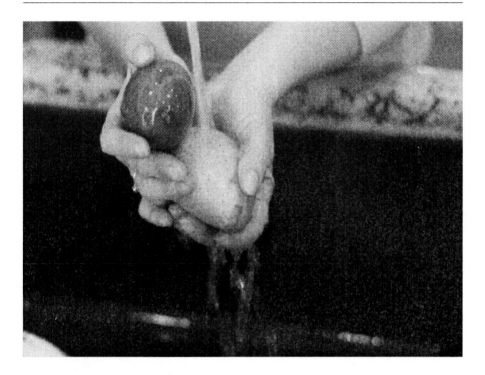

The Butyrate Paradox

Another paradox exists in the study of colorectal cancer called the "Butyrate Paradox." Butyrate is formed by intestinal microbes from highly-fermentable fiber residues, such as those from resistant starch, oat bran, pectin, and guar. Resistant starch consistently produces more butyrate than other types of dietary fiber but is largely missing from most diets, as are the other main butyrate producers. The role of butyrate in normal cells is completely different from its role in cancer cells—the butyrate paradox.

In normal colon cells, butyrate has an anti-inflammatory, health promoting effect. It has the opposite effect on cancer cells—butyrate causes cancer cells to self-destruct and die. Little is known about the signaling circuits that cause cancer cells to undergo apoptosis when exposed to butyrate. A recent hypothesis has been proposed:

> In a normal, healthy large intestine, butyrate is a preferred energy source. However, in the shortage of butyrate, attributed partly by "Western diet", glucose is substituted as the energy source for survival of these colonocytes. As they evolve to adapt to the new conditions, genetic manipulations are initiated with subsequent loss of function of critical genes and eventual loss of ability to undergo programmed cell death. These cells may therefore be considered as "normal" so that if the initial or healthy environment has been re-introduced, for example, by the presence of higher concentrations of butyrate, they will not be able to adapt rapidly due to their altered genetic make-up. Hence, they will undergo butyrate-induced apoptosis, as seen in many in vitro and animal studies.

In short, the answer to the butyrate paradox is to eat more resistant starch and other dietary fibers that produce butyrate. Without a steady supply of butyrate, colon cells turn to other fuels and don't behave normally. They lose their ability to self-destruct and turn cancerous. Normal cells self-destruct on a regular basis and when they are damaged, this keeps the colon health and cancer-free. A colon devoid of butyrate will soon become ill. A colon flooded with resistant starch will be happy and provide many years of trouble-free service.

The Carbohydrate Gap

Another major discrepancy in nutritional health science is found in our requirement for butyrate versus what the normal diet provides. Long-standing recommendations for 20-30 grams of fiber per day might be enough to produce all the butyrate we need if it all came from highly fermentable, butyrate producing fiber types but sadly it doesn't. The fiber in most people's diet is comprised of cellulose and plant cell walls, known as non-starch polysaccharides (NSP), and these produce very little butyrate. Oligosaccharides (OS), such as inulin and pectin, produce more butyrate than NSP, but are not found in large quantities in nature.

It's been calculated that we'd need to consume over 80 grams of fiber per day to meet our requirements for butyrate, and this is only if all of the fiber were highly fermentable. As discussed previously in the book, some of our ancestors appeared to have eaten over 130 grams of fermentable fiber daily—a feat that would be hard to match today. The 15-20 grams of dietary fiber that most people consume daily doesn't even account for 25% of the butyrate producing fiber we need, however, adding in 20-40 grams of RS would bridge this gap nicely.

Ancestral Precedents

Throughout the history of mankind, we enjoyed resistant starch. Whether by accident, luck or design, it's undeniable that RS is a big part of our past.

After we marched out of Africa, the first areas we settled were filled with palms. *Palmae* is one of the oldest plant families on earth and many early societies developed entire lifestyles in synergy with the various palm species:

- Date palm (Phoenix dactylifers) – Arabs of the sub-Saharan
- Palmyra palm (Borassus flabellifer) – Inhabitants of South India
- Lontar palm (Borassus sundaicus) – Roto islanders of Indonesia
- Coconut palm (Cocos nucifera) – Indo-Pacific Islanders
- Oil palm (Elaeis quineens) – West Africans
- Sago palm (Metroxylon sagu Rottboll) – Malaysians
- Moriche palm (Mauritia flexuosa) – American Paleo-Indians

What all of these palms had in common were amazing sources of fiber, particularly resistant starch. For instance, the Sago palm was the main source of subsistence throughout southern Asia until rice was introduced in 2500 BC. The sago palm is an amazing RS factory. In the first part of its life it looks like a short, trunk-less palm tree. When it is about 10 years old, it will send up a trunk 20-30 feet tall after which it flowers and dies. The year before it flowers, the large trunk is filled with up to 2000 pounds of easily extracted starch. The starch is unique in that it was easily isolated and dried, and when cooked and cooled, retrogrades into one of the most stable RS3 sources on the planet. Products made from sago starch can be stored for exceptionally long periods and helped the seafaring Malaysians travel far and wide throughout the Malay Archipelago. To this day, 25-40,000 tons of sago products are exported annually from Malaysia to the rest of the world.

One of the best sources of RS2 comes from the mountainsides of Asia. *Dioscorea opposita*, also known as Nagaimo, Japanese Mountain yam, Chinese yam, and Korean yam. It is often used in the Japanese noodle dish tororo udon/soba and as a binding agent in the batter of okonomiyaki. The grated nagaimo is known as tororo (in Japanese). In tororo udon/soba, the tororo is mixed with other ingredients that typically include tsuyu broth (dashi), wasabi, and green onions. Tororo is also eaten in China, Japan, Vietnam, Korea and the Philippines. Raw Chinese yam (*Dioscorea opposita*) is an excellent source of RS, as studied here:

> We examined the effects of raw Chinese yam (Dioscorea opposita), containing resistant starch (RS), on lipid metabolism and cecal fermentation in rats. Raw yam (RY) and boiled yam (BY) contained 33.9% and 6.9% RS, respectively...These results suggest raw yam is effective as a source of RS and facilitates production of short chain fatty acid (SCFA), especially butyrate.

Our past is filled with ample consumption of RS2, raw starch granules:

- *Horchata de Chufa*, a tiger nut starch drink that is still enjoyed by many around the world even today;
- *Fufu,* a starchy dough made from cassava root eaten in Africa;
- *Chicha*, similar to Horchata de Chufa but made with corn
- *Chuno*, a dehydrated potato staple of the Andes
- *Tororo*, made of the Asian yam *Dioscorea opposita*, often eaten with Natto
- Nuts and seeds, probably every single culture in the history of mankind has enjoyed munching on raw nuts and seeds. Sunflower seeds, pumpkin seeds, chia, flax, and all manner of tree and ground nuts are universally enjoyed by people around the world and contribute to a healthy gut.

Additionally, much evidence of RS3 consumption abounds:

- Yam cakes
- Dried, cooked tubers (ie. potato chips)
- Leftovers

It may be the "leftovers" that have given us our biggest supply of RS3 over the years. People living in so-called "Blue Zones" known for tremendous longevity are known to subsist on meager rations of leftover pasta and legumes.

Calorie counters rejoice!

When counting either total calories or carbohydrate calories, resistant starch is treated a bit differently. RS is not absorbed in the small intestine, therefore providing no direct energy (calories) to fuel your body. It is, however, converted into short-chain fatty acids in the large intestine. These fatty acids are either absorbed into the bloodstream or used by cells that line the colon as energy to fuel their activities.

Every 1 gram of RS is thought to provide approximately 1.5 calories (kcal) to the human body in terms of energy. Therefore, a daily intake of 40g RS would account for only 60 calories and should be counted as "fat" calories, not "carbs."

Towards a Daily Requirement

While there has been no official policy in the US or any other country, Australian officials are recommending a minimum of 20 grams of RS daily. Many of the studies we looked at used a range of 20-50 grams per day of RS to achieve the colon health and other aspects attributed to RS. No upper limit has been defined except in the case of excess gas or bloating noted by some study participants, but any excess starch consumed will simply pass through the entire digestive system undigested and harmlessly be eliminated.

In the absence of any official guidelines, I'd like to offer these:

- Eat daily from a selection of beans, rice, potatoes, bananas, plantains, sweet potatoes, squash, and other plants, roots, and tubers known to be rich in RS and inulin.
- Prepare your starchy foods in a way that will maximize the RS value, ie. cooking and cooling, raw or dried.
- For a supplement, use 1-2TBS of potato starch, Hi-Maize corn starch, or banana flour. Add it to a smoothie or just mix in water/yogurt. Most people find that 1-2TBS seems to be the sweet spot, but don't be afraid to try more or less. Many people like 4TBS a day, others 1 teaspoon. Find your own "sweet spot!"

When supplementing, start off slow, and work your way up. This gives your gut bugs time to get used to this new food source.

POTATO QUOTES

"ONE OF THE MAJOR DEVELOPMENTS IN OUR UNDERSTANDING OF THE IMPORTANCE OF CARBOHYDRATES FOR HEALTH IN THE PAST TWENTY YEARS HAS BEEN THE DISCOVERY OF RESISTANT STARCH."

— WORLD HEALTH ORGANIZATION, 1997

Notes:

CHAPTER 10. POTATO STARCH: A CRAZY WHITE POWDER THAT WENT VIRAL

While potato starch *is* resistant starch, I felt it deserved its own chapter in a book called *The Potato Hack*. Potato starch is a "hack" all its own, but a different type hack. Potato starch can be used as a dietary supplement to augment a diet low in fiber. I'm a huge fan of using potato starch as a prebiotic fiber supplement. Potato starch is found in the cooking aisle at your supermarket or on Amazon. There are organic varieties as well. All that's needed is a spoonful or two per day to give you all the fiber you need for healthy guts.

A couple of years ago I stumbled into what has been coined the "hack of the decade." No, not the potato hack, but the potato starch hack. I made the discovery that plain old potato starch, as commonly seen in supermarket baking aisles, is a second-to-none prebiotic, fermentable fiber. People all over the world are now using potato starch to improve their gut health.

This chapter is filled with ideas that have been common knowledge among scientists for nearly 30 years but have escaped the medical community and the general public until now. Resistant starch is recognized by dieticians, doctors, and much of the general public as a "thing," but they don't know what to do with it. People are more familiar with the term "fiber," but even that term has fallen out of favor as it has become more of a marketing gimmick than a health intervention.

Potato starch is a solution to many of our modern health woes—our electric, fast-paced lifestyle with its reliance on antibiotics and excessive sterilization has made us dependent on medications and makes us age faster than we should. Obesity, diabetes, and heart disease are killing us and placing a huge burden on the health care system and our personal finances. So many of our problems are brought on by diet alone and no one seems to realize or care. Potato starch can be part of the solution. Potato starch is a safe, concentrated form of resistant starch—easily sourced, cheap, and effective.

RS in the News and Journals

Around 2007, RS started making the news. Every so often, an article would pop up in a mainstream media news source saying that RS was a promising substance for improving health. These articles sometimes concluded that RS is found in potato salad, rice, and cornflakes. Just one problem, those sources of RS are very low in RS.

A 2007 study on pigs fed raw potato starch got me to thinking there were better sources of RS than potato salad:

OBJECTIVE:

The potential effect of a long-term intake of resistant starch on colonic fermentation and on gut morphologic and immunologic indices of interest in bowel conditions in humans was studied in pigs.

METHODS:

Sixteen growing pigs were meal fed for 14 wk on a diet containing a large amount of raw potato starch (RPS; resistant starch) or corn starch (CS; digestible starch). Effects were assessed in the colon from the physicochemical properties of digesta and in the intestinal morphology, including lymphocytic infiltration, apoptosis, and proliferation activities. Hematologic and blood leukocyte cell subsets analysis were performed.

RESULTS:

After 97 d, the digestive content from RPS pigs was heavier than for CS pigs, producing a hypertrophy of tunica muscularis. The proportion of butyrate was two-fold higher in proximal colon digesta in RPS pigs. RPS-fed pigs had reduced apoptosis in the crypts, lamina propria and lymphoid nodules in the colon, and ileal Peyer's patches. Fermentation of RPS reduced indices associated with damage to epithelial cells, such as crypt cell proliferation and magnesium excretion, whereas mucin sulfuration was increased, which promotes epithelial protection. The numbers of intraepithelial T cells and of blood leukocytes, neutrophils, and lymphocytes, mainly T-helper lymphocytes, were reduced in RPS pigs.

CONCLUSION:

Long-term intake of RPS induces pronounced changes in the colonic environment, reduces damage to colonocytes, and improves mucosal integrity, reducing colonic and systemic immune reactivity, for which health benefits in inflammatory conditions are likely to be associated.

[Cite: Nofrarías, M., Martínez-Puig, D., Pujols, J., Majó, N., & Pérez, J. F. (2007). Long-term intake of resistant starch improves colonic mucosal integrity and reduces gut apoptosis and blood immune cells. *Nutrition, 23*(11), 861-870.]

This study was eye-opening to me. When they fed pigs raw potato starch, their guts became super-"human". Pigs are often used in studies like this because their digestive systems are remarkably human-like and they can be dissected and studied in ways humans can't.

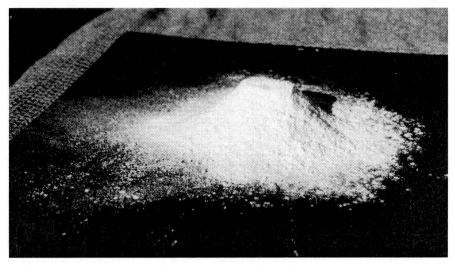

40 grams of Raw Potato Starch (Author's Photo)

This study was key for me. The pigs were fed *raw potato starch* but we were being told to eat *potato salad*. This may sound like reasonable advice, but it is not quite what it seems. Resistant starch is not all created equal. A raw potato contains RS type 2 and cooked and cooled potatoes contain RS type 3. RS2 is also found in green bananas, plantains, and cereal grains. It seemed to be the RS type 2 that was making the big changes in the pig intestines, but there are numerous studies in which RS2 and/or RS3 are fed to humans and it seems about 20-40 grams per day are needed to make big changes in health.

A couple of quick calculations show you'd need to eat about one raw potato or a couple of extremely green bananas a day to meet this goal if you wanted all RS2 from raw starch, of course you could try getting RS3 from cold potato salad, but it would take approximately 2-3 pounds to meet the need. If you are doing a 3 to 5-day potato hack, you are getting plenty of RS. But when you return to normal eating, you'll find RS is a bit hard to get.

Here's the dilemma: green bananas are terrible to eat, and raw potatoes are nearly as bad. Is all this worth eating 3 pounds of potato salad every day? You'd be fat as a pig if you did that! It just isn't that easy to get a lot of resistant starch in your diet.

There is an elegant solution, however. It's so simple that everyone who has ever read a study on RS that used raw potato starch as the vehicle for RS missed it: *raw potato starch is a common, cheap baking ingredient.*

Safety

This "hack" for great gut health couldn't be that easy. Something has to be wrong with it...surely you can't just buy a bag of cheap potato starch and expect it to work miracles in your broken, dyspeptic gut. But, it does seem to be as safe as any dietary intervention. There are some people for whom this may not be a great idea, and some for whom this trick may not work—I'll explain all that in a bit and give you some options. But plain ol' potato starch is a good start. It's not the be-all end-all for sure, but it has opened lots of eyes and caused quite a stir in certain circles. Let's take a look at all of the safety related concerns I've come up with so far.

The FDA's "Select Committee of 'Generally Recognized as Safe' Substances" issued a statement of the suitability of potato starch as a food item at the behest of none other than President Richard M. Nixon in 1969.

According to this special presidential committee:

> There is no evidence in the available information on unmodified potato starch that demonstrates or suggests reasonable grounds to suspect a hazard to the public...

and

> No adverse effects have been attributed to these starches as added food ingredients.

However, they did issue a couple of cautionary statements:

> Consumption of excessive quantities, pounds per day, of raw starch has resulted in obesity and iron-deficiency anemia in human subjects.

The Food and Drug Administration likewise did not see potato starch as a harmful substance as long as it was labelled correctly. They did not set a standard for potato starch because the US Pharmacopeia had already deemed potato starch safe and they deferred to them for safety concerns:

> In the absence of a standard of identity, starch meeting the specification of the United States Pharmacopeia is acceptable for food use.

USP Pharma Grade Potato Starch

The US Pharmacopeia, whose mission is to "…improve global health through public standards and related programs that help ensure the quality, safety, and benefit of medicines and foods," has deemed potato starch safe for inclusion in medicine and they've developed specifications for pharmacy-grade potato starch:

Potato Starch

Type of Posting	Notice of Adoption of Harmonized Standard
Posting Date	29–Feb–2012
Official Date	01–Dec–2012
Expert Committee	Monographs—Excipients

A harmonized standard for Potato Starch has been approved by the Pharmacopeial Discussion Group (PDG) as described in its PDG Sign-Off Cover Page. Having reached Stage 6 of the PDG process, the Potato Starch monograph has been formally approved by the USP Monographs—Excipients Expert Committee in accordance with the Rules and Procedures of the 2010–2015 Council of Experts.

Changes from the existing USP–NF monograph include:

* Updated acceptance criteria for Identification B to read "a thick opalescent" mucilage is formed consistent with PDG text, and to distinguish between other Starches.
* Updated Carbon Dioxide flow rate in Limit of Sulfur Dioxide test to be consistent with the text in the monograph and sign off text.
* Eliminated black diamond notation for Microbial Tests, as procedures are now fully harmonized within PDG.

The Potato Starch monograph will be incorporated into and become official with the Second Supplement to USP 35–NF 30.

As a food-grade item, potato starch is usually accompanied by a "Technical Data Sheet" from the supplier which look like this:

Technical data sheet:

* Appearance white powder moisture 20% max
* Whiteness 95.0 min
* Ph (30%suspension) 6.5-8.5
* Ash 0.25% max
* Sulphur dioxide (SO_2) 2ppm max
* Viscosity peak 1790b
* Granule size 150um (100 mesh sieve) 99.6% min

Sulfur Dioxide in Potato Starch

In all potato starch processing methods, an antioxidant is introduced at some point to keep the starch white. Commercially available starch is expected to be bright white and this is sometimes accomplished by adding sulfur dioxide. Sulfur dioxide is used widely in our food supply, if you are sensitive to sulfur dioxide, you may want to either make your own potato starch or find a raw starch that does not contain sulfur dioxide.

A review of dozens of technical data sheets from around the world showed that the sulfur dioxide contents ranged from less than 2ppm to 50ppm. The Food and Drug Administration issued a statement in 1976 concerning sulfur dioxide in food items:

> In view of the foregoing, the Select Committee concludes that: There is no evidence in the available information on ... sulfur dioxide that demonstrates, or suggests reasonable grounds to suspect, a hazard to the public when they are used at levels that are now current and in the manner now practiced.

Further, they indicated that sulfur dioxide is generally recognized as safe between 30-100 mg per kg of bodyweight. They estimate average intake is .2 to 2mg/kg of bodyweight (for 220-pound person, that's nearly 200mg per day).

The maximum SO2 content in potato starch, or 50ppm, would equate to 50 micrograms per gram of potato starch. Fifty grams of potato starch contains about 2.5 milligrams of SO2, at its highest noted concentration, which is well-below the FDA's limit of 200 milligrams per day for a 220-pound man.

Still, if you have a known sensitivity to sulfur dioxide, you may want to avoid potato starch. If you've ever had a reaction to foods that normally contain high levels of sulfur dioxide such as dried fruit, fruit juices, breakfast cereals, cookies, soft drinks, cereal bars, muesli bars, yogurt, ice cream, candy, frozen French fries, bread, margarine, or gluten-free flours, you may want to avoid potato starch. Sulfur dioxide may be especially troublesome for people with asthma.

Solanine in Potato Starch

A glycoalkaloid found naturally in potatoes, known as "Solanine," can be troublesome. Solanine is found in the leaves, sprouts, and green spots of potatoes and can be very toxic in large amounts—however it is not found in potato starch in measurable amounts. During the starch production process, the solanine is diluted and washed away with potato solids. Solanine may be found in effluents from potato starch factories and in the potato waste products generated during potato processing. Thirty to eighty percent of the solanine in the potato tuber are found in the outer layers. Thus, peeling greatly reduces solanine levels. The first step in the potato starch production process is washing and peeling the potatoes.

In commercially available potatoes, the solanine content is less than 20mg per kilogram. At this level, it is considered non-toxic, however, the solanine can accumulate in green spots and eyes...it's common-knowledge that these should be avoided. The National Institute of Environmental Health Sciences determined that the average consumption of solanine and other potato toxins was 12.75 mg glycoalkaloids per person per day, and that the lowest dose able to show toxic effects in humans is 5 times that at 1mg per kg of bodyweight, or about 50-70mg per day.

Potato Starch and Nightshade Allergy

Some people have "nightshade intolerances." Nightshade allergies stem from a malfunctioning immune system. Your body sees the proteins in potatoes (or other nightshades) as a harmful substance and attempts to fight them off. Your body immediately produces antibodies to destroy the nightshade proteins and these antibodies cause soft tissues throughout the body to become inflamed and swollen. Nightshade intolerance mainly affects the lungs, skin, and nasal passages and is seen as asthma, runny nose, watery eyes, scratchy/sore throat, sneezing, and possibly a rash. In severe cases, the lungs can swell leading to shortness of breath, chest pain and wheezing. Digestive symptoms are also common with any nightshade allergies. The intestinal tract can become inflamed from histamine, leading to vomiting, nausea, diarrhea, stomach cramping and abdominal pain.

Nightshade intolerances are presumably caused by the glycoalkaloids contained in nightshade plants (potatoes, peppers, eggplants, etc.) and linked to rheumatoid arthritis. One proven connection to the cause of these conditions is poorly diversified gut flora. Presumably, since the proteins are all removed, there should be no problems. But please err on the side of caution. If you've had allergic-type reactions to potatoes, peppers, eggplants, tomatoes, or pimentos, it's best you use a different raw starch—more on this in a bit.

Modified Potato Starch

Starch also has many non-food uses; it's used in glue, laundry spray, automotive and drilling industries, and many other obscure processing methods. Each one of these uses requires specially modified starch. If you suspect the potato starch you want to use is "modified" in any way—don't use it. A quick call to the manufacturer may be needed to be sure, but generally, if it's sold for food use, it's "unmodified." Below is a list of terms used when modifying potato starch, if you see any of these terms—don't use it:

- dextrin (E1400), roasted starch with hydrochloric acid
- alkaline-modified starch (E1402) with sodium hydroxide or potassium hydroxide
- bleached starch (E1403) with hydrogen peroxide
- oxidized starch (E1404) with sodium hypochlorite, breaking down viscosity
- enzyme-treated starch (INS: 1405), maltodextrin, cyclodextrin
- monostarch phosphate (E1410) with phosphorous acid or the salts sodium phosphate, potassium phosphate, or sodium triphosphate to reduce retrogradation
- distarch phosphate (E1412) by esterification with for example sodium trimetaphosphate, crosslinked starch modifying the rheology, the texture
- acetylated starch (E1420) esterification with acetic anhydride
- hydroxypropylated starch (E1440), starch ether, with propylene oxide, increasing viscosity stability
- hydroxyethyl starch, with ethylene oxide
- Octenyl succinic anhydride (OSA) starch (E1450) used as emulsifier adding hydrophobicity
- cationic starch, adding positive electrical charge to starch

- carboxymethylated starch with monochloroacetic acid adding negative charge

If you decide to use potato starch as a food item, it MUST be **unmodified**. It MUST be sold as a **food** item, generally purchased in a food aisle or website selling it as a **food-grade** item. If you suspect it is modified in any way—DON'T USE IT.

Potato Flour is NOT Potato Starch

Another product you may come across when looking for potato starch is potato flour—it's not the same thing. Potato flour is made from whole, cooked, and dried potatoes. It may look similar, but it contains very little resistant starch. Also beware of potato flakes—they are made from dehydrated, cooked potatoes, again no RS. These are not dangerous in any way; they are just not a source of RS. Use potato flour or flakes in recipes for taste and texture, but not for RS.

Amylose and Amylopectin

Potato starch is an amazing substance. One could literally spend a lifetime studying its properties and uses. It's multifaceted and simply amazing. Unimaginably complex yet incredibly simple.

Potato starch, like all starch, is composed of two types of starch: 80% amylopectin and 20% amylose. This starch is packed inside of granules that are spherical in shape that range from 10-100 micrometers across, averaging 36 micrometers—the largest of all starches. Potatoes use these starch granules to survive between growing seasons, turning the starch into sugars for energy and also to prevent themselves from freezing. These starch granules, known as amyloplasts, are specialized cells designed to store sugar in the form of starch.

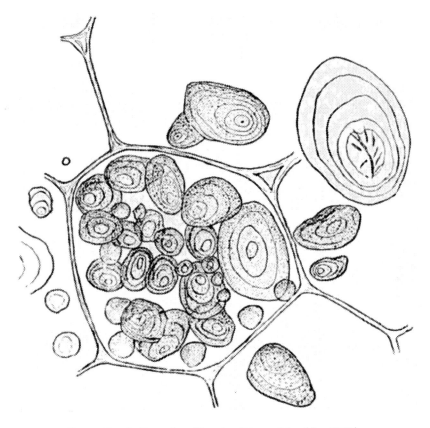

Potato Starch Granules, (Popular Science Monthly, 1899)

Inside of each starch granule's hard shell is a miniscule amount of water—20% by weight. When heated, this water swells and causes the starch granule to burst and turn into a sticky, gelatinous mess. This is the 'thickening' action that makes potato starch so sought after by cooks for gravies and sauces. As with everything about raw starch granules, this "little bit of water" is also not what it seems—it's not there by accident, it's an integral part of how starch works to provide energy for the plant. This water is highly purified and remains unfrozen even at − 30 degrees F. It's interspersed amongst the starch chains in a regular pattern and when looked at with an electron microscope, this pattern can be used to iden-tify the type of starch.

The amylose and amylopectin starches are works of art. The amylose starch is a helical spiral unit made up of glucose units.

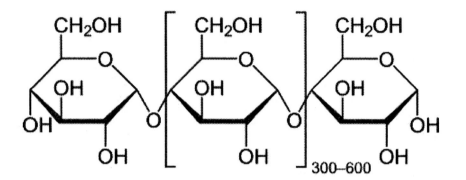

The amylopectin starch is made of the same basic building blocks, but is highly branched.

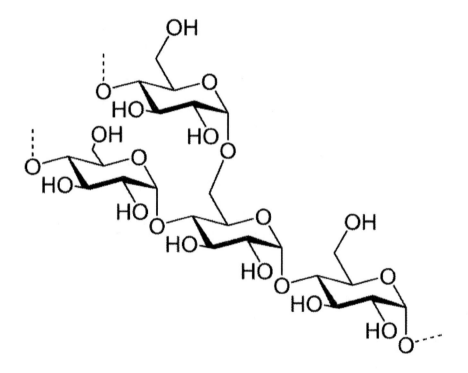

Prebiotic Potato Starch

When a human eats a raw potato, it gets broken down into tiny pieces through chewing and stomach actions. In the small intestine, the proteins and about 20% of the starch are digested. The remainder is termed "type 2 resistant starch," and serves as food for your gut microbes. This is *haute cuisine* for the bacteria in your intestines, something they evolved on for nearly 2 million years back when humans were more ape-like, but rarely see anymore. It's one of their favorite foods.

When a potato is heated and eaten, enzymes in our stomach and small intestine attack the ends of the amylose and amylopectin chains. Since the amylopectin starch is so highly branched, with lots of ends—it gets digested very fast. The amylose, with its tight bonds and only two ends, gets digested more slowly. A cooked potato with its two types of starch granules is really good food. It packs a punch in carbohydrates, protein, and even a bit of fat. It has a full complement of vitamins and minerals. It's good food...for us, but not our gut bugs. In fact, they go hungry on a meal of freshly cooked potatoes.

If the cooked potato is allowed to cool, the amylose and amylopectin starches undergo a process called retrogradation where the straight portions of each starch unit rejoin and form crystals. As the temperature drops, the crystals become tighter and tighter and the water which was inside them is expelled. This is why bread goes stale and stored potatoes turn dry. The retrogradation process begins at about 40 degrees F and is fully complete when the temperature drops to 17 degrees F. If you heat this potato back up, the retrograded starch actually gets stronger as more water is expelled. In fact, you can heat and cool it several times and with each cycle, more retrograded starch forms. When eaten, this provides a good meal for you AND your gut bugs. Win-win. This is the way humans cooked and ate for millions of years after we learned to cook food.

Adherence

When I was a kid on the farm, my mom used to make lots of home-made bread. A family favorite was a version called "Salt-Rising" bread. It differed from most breads in that it didn't need yeast to rise. The recipe called for putting a mixture of corn meal and potato slices in a bowl of warm water and keeping it warm for several days. This "starter" made our house smell like death, but the bread it produced covered any lingering smells and delighted us kids to no end. Here I am, 40 years later, finding out that mom's killer bread was the result of *potato magic*.

Raw potato starch granules have an amazing property in that they attract bacteria—both good and bad—and put it where it needs to go. This property, known as adherence, works through a mechanism known as "ligand mimicry." Animal and plant cells have receptors that allow for other cells to communicate with them, sometimes this inter-cell communication is the passing of hormones or transmitters that tell the cells to multiply or tell them to die. Drugs often target these receptor cells, as do pathogens and viruses. Anything that attaches to one of these receptors is known as a "ligand."

Potato starch is covered with receptors that do nothing except fool other cells into binding with them. This may seem inconsequential, but this exact same ligand mimicry is also seen in the fibers found in breast milk, known as Human Milk Oligosaccharides (HMOs). In human breast milk, there are hundreds of compounds called HMOs that serve as food for the baby's gut bugs. Any pathogenic microbe, and most non-pathogens, that encounters these HMOs will attach themselves to the HMOs—*and not the cells of the small intestine.* This prevents small bowel infections, diarrhea, etc... and is one reason why newborns are so bulletproof. Here's the point: ***Potato starch displays the same ligand mimicry as seen in HMOs.***

Potato starch can do two things for us with its little bag of tricks—it can take beneficial bacteria, for instance bifidobacteria, on a ride through the stomach and small intestine where bifidobacteria normally perish. It can "mop up" stray pathogens and viruses that are located in the stomach and small intestine, taking them to the large intestine where they can be dealt with by our body's defenses. In the case of cholera, a mixture of water and raw starches are given to the victim and recovery is rapid as the cholera leaves the small intestine and is eliminated. Unfortunately, most common pathogens like *Salmonella, Shigella, Klebsiella,* or *E. coli* do not bind. Although ligand mimicry does not sway these populations, the butyrate and SCFA generated improves intestinal ecology as well as lowers proliferation of these pathogens.

Potato Starch Processing Procedures

There are two places you can get potato starch—make it yourself or buy it in the store. As you may have guessed, I'm not a fan of overly processed foods such as wheat flour, vegetable oil, and high-fructose corn syrup. Some people are concerned that potato starch is somehow "unnatural," but that couldn't be further from the truth. Potato starch is a very natural product and found in large quantities in potatoes. A raw potato is about 20% starch by weight. A regular-sized potato (~1/2 pound) will yield about 40 grams of potato starch.

DIY Potato Starch

If you have the time and a few basic kitchen tools, you can easily make your own potato starch:

- Wash and peel 1 pound of firm Russet potatoes.
- Cut into cubes and place into an electric, centrifugal juice extractor.
- Collect the juice in a suitable pitcher or bowl.
- When the starch has mostly settled to the bottom, pour off as much liquid* as you can, leaving the settled starch undisturbed.
- Spread the wet starch onto a plastic or glass plate and allow to air dry overnight...a dehydrator on low heat would work even better.
- When the starch is thoroughly dried, you will find that you have collected approximately 4-6TBS (48-60 grams) of potato starch from a pound of potato.

*Potato juice is very healthy, too. Consider drinking the juice.

Starch Settling in Potato Juice (Author's Photo)

Commercial Potato Starch Extraction

Seeing how easy it was to extract starch at home simply by grating and squeezing, I wondered if store-bought potato starch was made as simply. I contacted a large manufacturer of potato starch and they gave me a look at how it's done on a large scale:

1. Freshly picked potatoes are placed in a rotating screen drum to remove any dirt, sand, or gravel.

2. The potatoes are blasted with very hot water and sent into a large vat of cold water where they are channeled and funneled towards a washing station.

3. At the washing station, the potatoes are rotated in another screen drum so that they agitate each other to remove any fungus, pesticides, or chemicals used in the growing process. They are blasted repeatedly with high pressure water to ensure complete cleanliness and to remove the peels.

4. The cleaned, peeled potatoes are sent into a rasper where they are finely ground into a slurry composed of starch, potato juice, and

potato pulp (protein and cell walls).

5. The potato slurry is sent to an extractor, a stainless steel, cone shaped, rotating drum, and blasted again with cold water to separate the starch from the other plant materials.

6. Sulfur dioxide is added at some point to prevent darkening of the starch, as previously discussed, this does not pose a health risk.

7. The crude "starch milk" that leaves the extractor gets sent to a refrigeration unit and is filtered and rinsed numerous times through smaller and smaller screens until all that remains is pure starch.

8. The final step is drying the moist starch in a flash dryer with hot air and sifting the starch one last time before packaging.

The only real difference between making your own potato starch and making it in an industrial setting is the use of sulfur dioxide. An industry paper shows that it is used at a rate of about 1 pound per ton of potatoes and carefully checked to ensure the amount found in the finished product is less than 50 parts per million, though more often it is less than 2ppm. Sulfur dioxide is used widely as a preservative in the processing of dried fruits and vegetables, and also in wine making. Sulfur dioxide is water soluble and is mostly gone from potato starch. However, if anyone is highly sensitive to sulfur dioxide, this may be a reason to avoid commercial potato starch and make your own instead.

RS Amounts in Potato

In many of the raw potato starch (RPS) studies, the researchers used 40 grams of resistant starch (RS) per day to achieve their goals of increased gut health. Here is a breakdown on the RS content in RPS and also in potatoes cooked in various ways, and even raw. Let's look at the nutrition label on a bag of potato starch.

We see that 1 tablespoon (TBS) of potato starch weighs 12 grams, and contains 10 grams of carbohydrate. The 20% disparity in weight vs. carbs makes sense since potato starch is 20% water. We also know that if we eat RPS, we won't be getting 10g of carbs—that is only effective for *cooked* potato starch. Studies show that RPS is between 65-85% RS, so we'll use 75%. 1TBS of RPS, therefore, should contain very close to 9 grams of RS (75% of 12 grams), and 4TBS will contain pretty close to 36g of RS.

If you are a chronic calorie counter, it is safe for you to figure that when eating uncooked RPS, you will not be getting the advertised 40 all-carbohydrate calories per tablespoonful. You will however get approximately 20 calories *from fat*. This seeming contradiction occurs because your gut bugs are the beneficiary of the eaten RPS, and they turn it into butyrate, a short-chain fatty acid (fat). Next, let's look at a potato.

Again, the nutrition data is always going to be for a cooked potato, but since we are going crazy here and throwing convention out the window, let's see what we can infer from the label as to its RS content when eaten raw.

The potato on the label weighs 148g, which would make it "three to the pound." This potato would be about the size of a tennis ball, for reference. Inside of its 148 grams of spud-licious goodness is a 20% starch content, give or take a few percent. If you had a machine that could wring out every last drop of starch, you'd find there were just under 30 grams of pure starch in this potato, or just under 3TBS. We know that pure potato starch is 75% RS2 by weight, so we can easily calculate that this potato, eaten raw, would provide us with 22 grams of RS.

Nutrition Facts

Serving Size 1 medium potato (148g/5.3 oz)

Amount Per Serving

Calories 110   Calories from Fat 0

	% Daily Value*
Total Fat 0g	0%
Saturated Fat 0g	0%
Trans Fat 0g	
Cholesterol 0mg	0%
Sodium 0mg	0%
Potassium 620mg	18%
Total Carbohydrate 26g	9%
Dietary Fiber 2g	8%
Sugars 1g	
Protein 3g	

Vitamin A 0%	•	Vitamin C 45%
Calcium 2%	•	Iron 6%

*Percent Daily Values are based on a 2,000 calorie diet. Your daily values may be higher or lower depending on your calorie needs:

	Calories:	2,000	2,500
Total Fat	Less than	65g	80g
Sat Fat	Less than	20g	25g
Cholesterol	Less than	300mg	300mg
Sodium	Less than	2,400mg	2,400mg
Potassium	Less than	3,500mg	3,500mg
Total Carbohydrate		300g	375g
Dietary Fiber		25g	30g

Calories per gram:
Fat 9 • Carbohydrate 4 • Protein 4

If instead of eating it raw, we decide to cook it and eat it hot, we'd find the RS content of this potato to be somewhere around .25 grams... not much. This measly amount is achieved because all of the "resistance" cooked out of the starch—it is now considered "readily digestible starch," good for you but nothing for your gut bugs. Potato starch gelatinizes, that is, the starch granules swell and burst—destroying the RS2 value when the starch reaches about 140 degrees F.

Taking it all a step further, let's cool this guy down. We'll put him in our refrigerator overnight and chill him right down to about 35 degrees. The next morning, we find that the readily digestible starch has retrograded into a bit of RS—it now has about 3.5 grams of RS3. We'll keep going and chop this potato into cubes and heat it up in a hot pan with a bit of oil to brown it nicely. At this point, our poor, reheated potato will have about 4 grams of RS3. Cool it down again, 4.5 grams of RS3. Heat it back up—5 grams, cooled again—5.5 grams, reheated—6g. Eventually it will stop, but what I wanted you to see was how the biggest boost in RS was at the very first cooling and reheating cycle. After that, it lessens.

To recap:

1 medium potato, tennis ball sized, 150g or so, can be looked at like this in terms of resistant starch:

- Raw – 22g
- Cooked – .25g
- Cooled – 3.5g
- Re-heated – 4g
- Re-cooled – 4.5g
- Re-re-heated – 5g
- Re-re-cooled – 5.5g
- Re-re-re-heated – 6g

Measuring RS

Resistant starch in foods is officially measured with a standardized test protocol known as AOAC 2002.02. This test was adopted in 2002 by the Association of Agricultural Chemists to ensure accurate reporting of RS contents. Test labs that measure RS using AOAC 2002.02 cannot measure any values higher than about 64% RS by weight, and all measures of potato starch via this protocol result in an RS value of 64%. Potato starch contains the highest level of RS of any natural (or synthetic) starch.

Potato Starch as an RS Supplement

Potato starch is a good way to boost resistant starch consumption to a level close to what was being used in human studies to good effect.

Here are some noteworthy scientific studies using raw, unmodified potato starch in varying amounts:

- Langworthy et al. described bloating and discomfort with 180g of raw potato starch and none with 60g. It was also noted that when human subjects were fed over 40g of potato starch, a portion was found in feces, indicating that microbiome may only be able to process up to 40g of potato starch in a single feeding (Langworthy, 1920).

- 17-30g/day of raw potato starch in 15-day human trials increased SCFA (Aller, 2011).

- Three separate studies show that the prebiotic effects of raw potato starch are as, or more, effective than RS from other sources. Raw potato starch is a preferred substrate by bifidobacteria over starches from pea and wheat. That when compared with wheat or barley starches, potato starch induced greater amounts of satiety and postprandial glucose control and was on par with experiments measuring lipid metabolism, glucose control, and insulin response. When compared with maize, wheat, and pea starch raw potato starch provided more butyrate than other starches studied (Wronkowska, 2009).

- Raw potato starch increased short chain fatty acid production and enhanced the proportion of butyrate. Raw potato starch increased fecal weight and shortened transit time slightly (Ferguson, 2000).

- 50g of raw potato starch created less hydrogen than 10g of lactulose indicting it was being fermented in the large intestine by a different population of microbes that digest sugars (Burge, 2000).

- Raw potato starch was compared to FOS. It was found that raw potato starch is fermented mostly in the caecum and proximal colon, where FOS was fermented distally. However, with the raw potato starch, more lactate was produced distally. This study shows why raw potato starch on its own may not be as beneficial as raw potato starch combined with other fiber sources (LaBlay, 2003).

- Raw potato starch significantly increased absorption of calcium and magnesium without altering plasma levels. When inulin was added, the effect was even better (Mineo, 2009).
- Adding 50g of raw potato starch to a human diet reduced postprandial glycemia and insulinemia (Higgins, 2014).
- Raw potato starch reduced the large intestine damaging effects of a high protein diet (Birt, 2013).
- Raw potato starch stimulated the growth of bifidobacteria and lactobacteria as well as short chain fatty acids which were found to be useful for the suppression of pathogenic organisms in the colon (Barczynska, 2015).

References:

Aller, E. E., Abete, I., Astrup, A., Martinez, J. A., & Baak, M. A. V. (2011). Starches, sugars and obesity. *Nutrients, 3*(3), 341-369.

Barczyńska, R., Śliżewska, K., Libudzisz, Z., Kapuśniak, K., & Kapuśniak, J. (2015). Prebiotic properties of potato starch dextrins. *Advances in Hygiene & Experimental Medicine/Postepy Higieny i Medycyny Doswiadczalnej, 69.*

Birt, D. F., Boylston, T., Hendrich, S., Jane, J. L., Hollis, J., Li, L., ... & Schalinske, K. (2013). Resistant starch: promise for improving human health. *Advances in Nutrition: An International Review Journal, 4*(6), 587-601.

Burge, M. R., Tuttle, M. S., Violett, J. L., Stephenson, C. L., & Schade, D. S. (2000). Potato-lactulose breath hydrogen testing as a function of gastric motility in diabetes mellitus. *Diabetes technology & therapeutics, 2*(2), 241-248.

Ferguson, L. R., Tasman-Jones, C., Englyst, H., & Harris, P. J. (2000). Comparative effects of three resistant starch preparations on transit time and short-chain fatty acid production in rats. *Nutrition and cancer, 36*(2), 230-237.

Higgins, J. A. (2014). Resistant starch and energy balance: impact on weight loss and maintenance. *Critical reviews in food science and nutrition, 54*(9), 1158-1166.

Langworthy, C. F., & Deuel Jr, H. J. (1920). Digestibility of raw corn, potato and wheat starches. *J. Biol. Chem, 42*, 27-40.

Le Blay, G. M., Michel, C. D., Blottiere, H. M., & Cherbut, C. J. (2003). Raw potato starch and short-chain fructo-oligosaccharides affect the composition and metabolic activity of rat intestinal microbiota differently depending on the caecocolonic segment involved. *Journal of applied microbiology, 94*(2), 312-320.

Mineo, H., Ohmi, S., Ishida, K., Morikawa, N., Machida, A., Kanazawa, T., ... & Noda, T. (2009). Ingestion of potato starch containing high levels of esterified phosphorus reduces calcium and magnesium absorption and their femoral retention in rats. *Nutrition research, 29*(9), 648-655.

Wronkowska, M., Soral-Śmietana, M., & Krupa-Kozak, U. (2009). Native wheat, potato and pea starches and their physically modified preparations tested in vitro as the substrates for selected Bifidobacterium strains. *International journal of food sciences and nutrition, 60*(sup4), 191-204.

Alternatives to Potato Starch

If you cannot tolerate potato starch, there are viable alternatives. It may also be a good idea to "change things up" every now and then just to keep your gut bugs guessing. It's doubtful our ancestors ate the same things day-in and day-out so there's no reason for us to either.

The cooked food portions of resistant starch are fairly easy—get your RS3 from cooked and cooled potatoes, rice, beans, and the other sources. For RS2, the raw starch granules, you'll need to be a little pickier. Other sources of RS2 equivalent to potato starch can be found in green banana or plantain flour, high-amylose corn starch, or tapioca starch. A brief description of each follows:

Banana Flour

All bananas, which include plantains and "dessert" bananas, start out green, hard to peel, and filled with raw starch granules that are resistant to digestion and an excellent source of RS2. As bananas ripen, they turn yellow and the RS2 quickly converts to sugar.

A very delicious flour is made around the world from green bananas, most often the plantain variety, and makes a suitable substitute for gluten containing flours in baked goods. What's even better, when eaten raw, banana flour is a potent source of RS2. The RS content in banana flour is a bit less than in potato starch because the starch is not extracted, the entire banana is dried and ground. Even so, the RS content is a respectable 50% by weight.

In some ways, banana flour is even better for us than potato starch in that it contains all the nutrients, vitamins, and plant fibers found in the original fruit. This distinction is very important and makes banana flour a very desirable source of RS2.

Tapioca Starch

Tapioca is made from the extracted starch of the cassava plant. While the raw starch of the cassava has been noted to be very high, up to 80%, in fact, the isolated starches have come in with mixed results. Some studies that measured the RS in tapioca starch found as little as 5% and as much as 50%. The differences are due to the species of cassava used and also possibly the processing methods. Until more is known, tapioca starch should be used with caution as an RS source.

Corn Starch

Regular corn starch used in cooking contains very little RS, maybe 2-3% by weight. There is another type of corn starch known as high-amylose starch which is made from specially bred corn containing up to 55% RS2. In many of the studies done on RS health benefits, this corn starch is called "HAMS" for High Amylose Maize Starch. HAMS is available commercially as HI-Maize cornstarch.

Other starches –

There are several other starches that have great promise as RS2 sources. Mung bean starch, buckwheat starch, and pea starch all show high levels of RS2, but no studies have been done to catalog the RS remaining in commercially available products. Hopefully one day, these starches will come with a label showing the exact RS content, but until then use at your own discretion.

Hopefully you read this chapter as it was intended, a simple treatise on the beauty and simplicity of potato starch as a suitable supplement for resistant starch. The science behind potato starch is simply fascinating and the scientific/medical experimentation which has been performed just adds to the mystique. If and how you use potato starch is completely up to you, but our sincere hope is that you don't discard all the other advice I've given you and jump straight into high doses of potato starch in an attempt to turn around years of medical issues and poor lifestyle or dietary choices. Potato starch may very well be the one item that tips things in your favor, or it may end up being something you don't need, only you will be able to decide. If, one day, you begin to see row after row of miracle resistant starch supplements, please keep in mind that plain ol' potato starch can be just as good.

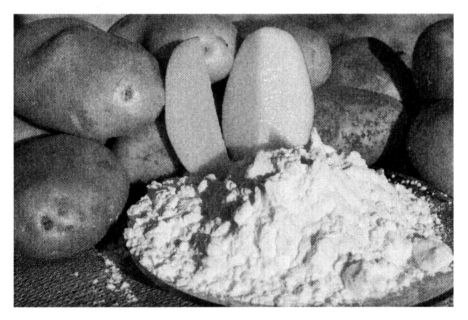

Potato Starch (Author's Photo)

POTATO QUOTES

"A gem is not polished without rubbing, nor a man perfected without potatoes."

- Irish Saying

Notes:

Chapter 11. The Human Gut Microbiome

The potato hack is predominantly a hack on your gut. When you eat only potatoes for a few days the bacteria in your gut evolve quickly and pass their genes back and forth. Hundreds of thousands of generations of bacteria will thrive in those few days that you are eating only potatoes. This rapid evolution creates an environment not seen in your gut since you were a breastfed baby. During the potato hack it is quite likely that your gut is healthier than it has been since you were a toddler.

So many times it's said that the human gut microbiome is just too complicated, too massive, and just "is." People liken the micro-inhabitants of our guts with our autonomous nervous system...a real entity but one which we have no control over. This couldn't be further from the truth.

The multitudinous combinations of microbes that can inhabit a human contribute to our genetic individuality and our resistance (or propensity) to disease. The genetically diverse microbiome is, as predicted by Hippocrates thousands of years ago, the major driver in our health. The gut controls digestion, nutrition, inflammation, sleep, mood, growth, immunity, and more. We, the host, control how the microbes are fed and housed and in turn, their overall numbers and diversity. Until recently we didn't have this luxury. As we learn more about our microbiome through modern test methods we get closer and closer to being able to manipulate our microbiome with pinpoint accuracy.

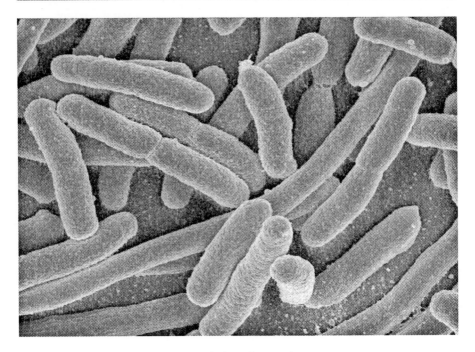

E. coli (Pixabay.com)

Throughout the book I discuss the human microbiome as a simple concept. The truth is, though, the reality of our gut is more complex than anyone can really fathom. Yet it is so elegantly simple it should require no thought whatsoever. Modern life is tough on our guts. Nature saw fit to give us 100 trillion helpers to see us through life and we fritter and waste them in an off-hand way. Let's get to know our microbiome and learn to conduct the orchestra rather than being a casual observer.

Taxonomy 101 (Run!)

Welcome to your worst nightmare. A whole chapter on biology...it's 11th grade all over again. If you are one of those strange ducks that actually loved high school biology, maybe even going on to get an advanced degree, you will be in heaven! For the other 99.9% of humankind, I'm going to try to make this as painless as possible.

We are living in amazing times...more is known now about the trillions of microbes in our gut than ever before. Not only do we know more about them, but can see them and we even know how to influence them. Until recently, the gut microbiome was something we loved to hate because we focused on disease, the unwanted pathogens. Our gut microbiome was once 'the great unknown' and considered a confounder in all disease.

Doctors routinely destroy their patients' intestinal microbiome over the most superfluous sickness. Toddlers' ear infections are blasted with round after round of antibiotics. We have been led to believe we need to use 'household napalms' to kill off 99.999% of all germs.

As more and more people get their gut microbes tested, we learn even more. Already we are seeing theories on gut bugs topple as person after person disproves the standing theories. For example, it was long thought that a gut bug called Akkermansia was the "anti-obesity" microbe. Believe it or not, people were begging for Akkermansia probiotics to lose weight. Now we discover that Akkermansia possibly causes weight loss by stealing nutrients and degrading protective mucous coatings in the gut often leading poor health.

This chapter will be the one you need to bookmark. If you decide to get your gut microbes tested through one of the many new companies that offer this amazing new service, you will want to read and re-read this chapter. I apologize in advance if this chapter gives you the hives or causes flashbacks to the halcyon days of your youth. Please have a read through. Rest assured, there will be no test at the end—the test is going to be the rest of your life.

FANCY CHARTS & BIG WORDS, $99, please

There are currently three or four companies that offer testing of intestinal microbes. Some require a prescription from a doctor, some don't. Some will contain detailed information related to specific bacterial species, pathogens, and other markers of health. Others will just give you some basic information about the major types of gut bugs present. If you decide to get one of these tests, it may behoove you to get familiar with some of the terminology used and how to interpret the results you get back.

Here is a list of terms associated with sampling gut microbes:

• 16S rRNA
• 18S rRNA
• Shotgun metagenomics
• Illumina sequencing
• .fasta files
• Basic Local Alignment Search Tool, or **BLAST**
• MG-RAST

I figured the quickest way to chase readers away would be to give a detailed description of each one of these terms. Instead, here's the gist: Really smart people with really expensive laboratory equipment have figured out how to look at a sample of your poop and figure out what lives in your gut. All you need to be concerned about is the report they send you. Talk to others, find a company that fits your financial means and specializes in the information you seek. If you are just curious, get a test that shows a comprehensive list of microbes. If you are ill, you'll want to work with a doctor to get a test that shows pathogens as well. Gut bug testing 'just for fun' may just be one of the biggest indulgences mankind has ever been afforded. Bear in mind, the report you get for $99 today would have cost millions of dollars just 10 years ago.

What you'll notice first off in your report are lots of long names like Ruminococcaceae or *Bifidobacterium*. Some of these long words are in italics, some are not. There is no rhyme or reason behind this. I think that sometimes it makes the person who compiles the report feel smarter than everybody else. Or they are just making it up as some kind of cruel joke. Either way—*it doesn't matter.* Later on I'll go into some detail about specific microbes and what they do.

In your report there may be names of bacteria that were found in your poop sample but really shouldn't be there. Many of these, known as pathogens or opportunists, are a normal part of a healthy gut ecosystem, but if they grow out-of-control, they cause big trouble and will require intervention. Some are never supposed to be there. Let's hope your report is sufficiently accurate and thorough to identify these.

There are probably only three reasons to send off for one of these reports—curiosity, doctor's orders, or self-diagnosis. Here's how to handle each scenario:

Curiosity

Many people have become interested in what's in their guts because they've read some of the thousands of articles on the importance of gut bacteria. If you decide to get a test done of your stool, the best way to handle the report is as if you had the eyes of a child...look, read, and take it all in. Then, get yourself to Google and start searching for the listed microbes. Make a report, save the links you use, send it to all your geeky friends or bloggers who love this stuff. You will be amazed to find you may have gut bugs that are normally only found in cows or sheep, or ones found normally in fish. If you are healthy and happy to begin with, don't let this report change you! Nothing contained in this report predicts the end of the world as you know it. Maybe you can see right off you lack many gut bugs that others have or you have ones nobody else does. If your diet is terrible and you need a reason to clean it up—maybe this will give you the motivation you need. Use your gut report as your introduction to your intestinal microbiome—not as a way to diagnose and treat major medical conditions.

This can be a fun hobby, if you have the time, money, and inclination I highly recommend seeing what type of bacteria inhabit your intestines. The more testing that people do, the bigger the libraries of identified bacteria become. This is citizen science at its finest.

Doctor's Orders

If you are under medical supervision for a gut related illness, or if your doctor orders a test of your gut microbes, ask for a copy of the results. These reports will be more detailed than the other consumer type reports, and in some ways less useful to the curiosity seeker. It won't look as nice, it will be harder to read, but that's OK. Your doctor will know what to do with the report and the information it contains.

If you have any doubts, get a second opinion. If you trust your doctor, follow their advice and recommendations to the letter. Don't use the doctor's report to go out and treat yourself. Nothing will mess things up faster than a patient 'going rogue' against their doctor's orders. In fact, you could make the situation much worse.

Self-diagnosis of Illnesses

This is a valid reason to get one of these advanced gut microbiome reports, but it could potentially be the most dangerous. If you've suffered a life of gastrointestinal illnesses and think that maybe your doctor is "behind the times," find one of the non-prescription labs that test gut bacteria and see what you find. Do like the others with your report—spend some quality time on the internet, make a report, and satisfy your curiosity. If you see any huge red flags, you can go one of two routes: fix yourself or ask for a doctor's help. If you see tons of pathogens and harmful parasites—see a doctor. If you see minor abnormalities compared to others, talk it out at gathering places like forums or blogs where this is the topic of the day.

The modern gut is generally not healthy, but if you have relatively few complaints and an uninterested doctor, self-treatment may be your only option. So many people are eating wrong—wrong for themselves and especially wrong for their gut bugs. If your goal is self-diagnosis, I'd suggest buying several test kits. Make a few changes and re-test. This may get a bit expensive, but it may be well worth it. After each change you make, wait 3-6 months before retesting. It takes time for gut bugs to adjust to new settings. If you think you see big problems, take the report and go see a doctor.

King Philip Eats What?

Here's another thing you'll notice on your report or when you start searching the internet for descriptions, there will be a laundry list of Phyla. If you can remember back to Biology 101, you'll maybe remember the little ditty: 'King Philip Came Over For Good Spaghetti' or 'King Philip Curses Out Funky Green Salad'. King Philip, whoever that is, must have known a lot about biology. Certainly more than most of the students who required these silly mnemonics to remember the order of these words:

- Kingdom
- Phylum
- Class
- Order
- Family

- Genus
- Species

When you see this laundry list of gut microbiome Phyla (singular form of Phylum—again, makes no sense), don't be too concerned. The laundry list of gut bugs I refer to is this:

- Firmicutes
- Bacteriodetes
- Proteobacteria
- Actinobacteria
- Verrucomicrobia
- Tenericutes
- Cyanobacteria
- Fusobacteria

A good report on your gut bugs is going to contain a section on the relative percentages of these Phyla. This is good information to look at quickly. You can point to the pretty colors used in making the pie chart. Exhale a few hmmmmm's and ohhhhhh's, but only to impress your spouse who thinks you just wasted your money.

CSI TAXONOMY, or, Who's Getting in my Trash at Night?

If you had a problem with animals getting into your trash cans at night, you might hire ACME Exterminators to stake out your back yard. Would you be happy with a report the next day that says:?

"We have positively identified the marauders as *Chordata*."

The first thing you'd notice is the italics. Next, you'd pay any amount of money in the world to get the *Chordata* off your property. Anything in *ITALICS* has to be *bad*. If you had a computer and an internet connection, as many people have nowadays, you could search for the word *Chordata*. You won't even need to put it in italics! The computer doesn't care. The first result you find for *Chordata*:

"Chordates (Chordata) are a group of animals that includes more than 75,000 living species. Chordates are divided into three basic groups: vertebrates, tunicates, lancelets. Of these, the vertebrates—lampreys, mammals, birds, amphibians, reptiles and fishes—are the most familiar and are the group to which humans belong."

Huh? You just paid good money to learn that a creature with a backbone was in your yard? Maybe your spouse is right—-this is a waste of money after all.

Not entirely. In your intestines are between 500 and 1,000 different species of gut bugs. These hundreds of species will fall under the eight different phyla listed above. Knowing some common relationships can help you understand how well your gut is populated with the microbes that keep you healthy and the microbes that make you sick.

Also on the report, should be several different families, genera, species and sub-species. Most people do not know if these words are singular or plural, and again, it *doesn't matter*. Once you know the family, you can at least be assured that a canine was getting in your trash. Knowing the genus could tell you this canine was a dog. Once you discover the species and sub-species, for instance, you can now walk across the street to Mr. Jeffrey's house and demand he keeps little Barney the beagle out of your trash.

It's the same thing with your gut bugs.

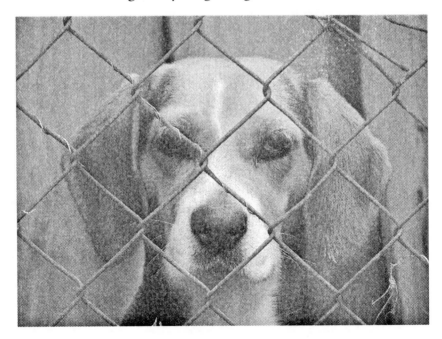

Bad, Chordata, Bad! (Pixabay.com)

So, Who's in my Gut, Anyway?

For your future reference, here is a list of the major Phyla and what each is thought to contribute to your intestinal microbiome:

Firmicutes

(Latin: *firmus*, strong, and *cutis*, skin, referring to the cell wall) are a phylum of bacteria, most of which have Gram-positive cell wall structure. A few, however, such as *Megasphaera*, *Pectinatus*, *Selenomonas* and *Zymophilus*, have a porous pseudo-outer-membrane that causes them to stain Gram-negative. They have round cells, called cocci or rod-like forms. Many Firmicutes produce endospores, which can survive extreme conditions. Firmicutes make up the 'compost pile' in your guts—they love to eat plant matter, both inside and outside your body. It's Firmicutes that give that pile of old leaves its wonderful smell and also the group that makes your expensive wine go sour. Some strains of *Lactobacillus* and other lactic acid bacteria are Firmicutes and may possess potential therapeutic properties including anti-inflammatory and anti-cancer activities. They are found in various environments, and the group includes some notable pathogens—such as Anthrax and Tetanus. This phylum generally makes up 20-75% of most people's gut microbiome...it's a large phylum with hundreds of different genera. It's also very diet, age, and geography related. Don't worry too much about the size of your Firmicutes.

Bacteroidetes

Composed of three large classes of Gram-negative, non-spore-forming, anaerobic, and rod-shaped bacteria that are widely distributed in the environment, including in soil, sediments and seawater as well as in the guts and on the skin of animals. Members of the genus *Bacteroides* are opportunistic pathogens. Rarely are members of the other two classes pathogenic to humans. Bacteriodetes are the second major phylum in your gut. Don't be surprised if they account for nearly half of all your microbes. These microbes are voracious eaters and will happily eat anything you give them, producing in return, gasses and smells galore. A well-nourished gut will be full of less noxious Bacteriodetes than a gut starved of its more preferred foods, such as plant fiber and resistant starches.

Proteobacteria

Includes a wide variety of pathogens, such as *Escherichia, Salmonella, Vibrio, Helicobacter,* and many other notable genera. Carl Woese established this grouping in 1987, calling it informally the "purple bacteria and their relatives". Because of the great diversity of forms found in this group, the Proteobacteria are named after Proteus, a Greek god of the sea capable of assuming many different shapes. If your report shows a relatively high percentage of Proteobacteria, it could be an indication that you need a diet overhaul or lifestyle changes (quit smoking, start exercising). These microbes are associated with inflammation, but they are not a death-sentence. In fact, many of these types of gut bugs are necessary for producing certain chemicals used in digestion.

Actinobacteria

A group of Gram-positive bacteria. They can be terrestrial or aquatic. Although known primarily as soil bacteria, they are actually more abundant in freshwaters. Actinobacteria is one of the dominant bacterial phyla. Actinobacteria are mainly all "good guys." These bacteria produce antibiotics and are excellent decomposers of plant matter. Bifidobacteria belong to this phylum and are some of the most sought-out microbes as they have been identified as "super-bugs" for human health.

Verrucomicrobia

A recently described phylum of bacteria. This phylum contains only a few described species. The species identified have been isolated from freshwater and soil environments and human feces. Evidence suggests that verrucomicrobia are abundant within the environment, and important (especially to soil cultures). Though not very abundant, their presence indicates a well-balanced microflora. These may be more important to other microbes than to you. Excessive cleanliness and sterilising every morsel you eat is a reason for a lack of Verrucomicrobia—playing in the mud and eating veggies that are a bit dirty is the best way to attract these gut bugs.

Tenericutes

These lack a cell wall and therefore are Gram negative. Notable genera include the Mycoplasma, Ureaplasma and Phytoplasma. These are found in very low number in gut microbiomes, but important nonetheless. They are found in the guts of most mammals and can be either completely harmless or extremely pathogenic—they have been implicated in pneumonia, bronchitis, other respiratory illnesses and infertility.

Cyanobacteria

A phylum of bacteria that obtain their energy through photosynthesis. The name "cyanobacteria" comes from the blue color of the bacteria. Not much is known about these and what they may or may not do for us. These bacteria are the hardiest in the world, being found in the world's most extreme environments such as deep-sea sulfur vents and on the bare rocks of Antarctica. They are referred to as 'blue-green algae' when found as scum in polluted water.

Fusobacteria

A rod-shaped Gram-negative bacteria. Found commonly in the intestines of all animals, some are good, some are bad. These will barely register on most people's reports if at all.

What constitutes a "good" gut microbiome then?

What does a good gut microbiome look like, or is there even a "perfect" gut profile? With the advent of modern testing, scientists have scoured the world looking at the gut flora of different populations and they've discovered that gut flora is as diverse as people. Healthy kids in Africa have a much different gut flora than healthy kids in Europe, and we all know baby guts look much different from those of toddlers and adults. So what gives? How can people with such diverse looking guts all be equally healthy? Gut bugs that are doing a great job have some things in common and unhealthy people have similarities in their guts that also shouldn't be overlooked.

Additionally, most gut testing completely misses the friendly (or not-so-friendly) fungi present in a human. It's been supposed that quite possibly the yeast and fungus present in a human gut (the "mycobiome") is of more importance than the bacteria present.

The health of any community may really just come down to its stability. This applies equally to nations, families, herds of animals, forests, and even gut microbiomes. Frederik Blakhed, in a recent review of the gut microbiome wrote:

> A healthy microbiome, considered in the context of body habi-
> tat or body site, could be described in terms of ecologic stabil-
> ity (i.e., ability to resist community structure change under stress
> or to rapidly return to baseline following a stress-related change),
> by an idealized composition or by a desirable functional profile
> (Blakhed, 2012, *Defining a healthy human gut microbiome: current con-
> cepts, future directions, and clinical applications.*)

In the review, he surmised that a healthy gut biome, just like a healthy
nation or state, needs to display "resistance" and "resilience." In other
words, a healthy gut biome will resist change and also bounce back after
an incident that upsets it. The concept that a healthy microbial community can be defined by certain percentages of bacterial phyla is just too
simplistic based on the huge differences seen between healthy people.

Resistance and resilience in a gut ecology is disrupted when the microbes contained in it become less diverse, as after rounds of antibiotics.
These altered gut microbiomes cannot fight off pathogens such as C. Diff
and other opportunistic bacteria which would normally be kept in check
by a resistant gut flora.

People may get by for a long time, in fact, most people nowadays
have less-than-stellar gut floras thanks to our modern reliance on antibiotics, genetically engineered crops with built-in bug killers, and poor
diets. This doesn't mean we will all succumb to cancer and other diseases
of the day, but it does mean that we don't have a gut biome that is actively
fighting these things off, either.

Re-POOP-ulating the Gut

In 2013, researchers from Ottawa devised the perfect blend of bacteria to re-POOP-ulate the guts of people who were experiencing recurrent C-Diff infections that didn't respond to normal treatment. Similar to
a fecal transplant, this team isolated 33 different microbes from a healthy
donor, grew the microbes in test tubes, and implanted living, thriving
colonies directly into the recipient's large intestine. Within 2 days, the
patients fully recovered and led normal lives for the 6 months of follow-
up done. Their recipe for re-COLON-ization?

- Acidaminococcus intestinalis
- Bacteroides ovatus
- Bifidobacterium adolescentis
- Bifidobacterium longum
- Blautia producta
- Clostridium cocleatum
- Collinsella aerofaciens
- Dorea longicatena
- Escherichia coli
- Eubacterium desmolans
- Eubacterium eligens
- Eubacterium limosum
- Eubacterium rectale
- Eubacterium ventriosum
- Faecalibacterium prausnitzii
- Lachnospira pectinoshiza
- Lactobacillus casei
- Parabacteroides distasonis
- Raoultella
- Roseburia faecalis
- Roseburia intestinalis
- Ruminococcus torques
- Ruminococcus obeum
- Streptococcus mitis

The Namur Treasure

Namur, Belgium, 1996. A sealed oak barrel was discovered in a Middle Age archeology site. After much speculation as to the treasure trove of information contained in this time capsule, it was pried open under the watchful eye of scientists...what lied within? Gold, maps, ancient texts? No, better! A big old Middle Age turd! A not just any old turd, this was a beauty...a 121.4 gram, dark-brown, well-preserved specimen given the number Z04F56 and deposited into a storage facility in Marseille, France.

In 2007, Z04F56 was unceremoniously exhumed from storage, its outer layers peeled back, and its inner-most secrets revealed. Microscopic examination revealed the suspected plant fibers, pollens, and seeds but also eggs of parasites Trichuris trichiura and Acanthamoeba two very common human-infective, swine-transmitted, pathogens. 16S rRNA sampling of the "Treasure of Namur" showed a highly diverse gut flora, many rarely seen species such as Paenibacillus macerans, Bacillus jeotgali, Staphylococcus pasteuri, Staphylococcus epidermidis, Staphylococcus cohnii, Micrococcus luteus, Pseudomonas geniculata, Stenotrophomonas maltophilia, Bacillus horti and Clostridium magnum were identified. Also Rhodanobacter, Paenibacillus, Paenibacillus macerans, Paenibacillus thiaminolyticus, Paenibacillus ehimensis, Staphylococcus arlettae, Propionibacterium acnes and Enterobacter cloacae. While this list may not seem impressive to the untrained eye, to researchers it is a gold-mine of information. This ungainly remnant of the Middle Ages gives clues to the diversity of a gut flora long since "passed."

Hitchhiker's Guide to the Gut

Throughout this book I use several terms interchangeably...gut and intestine mean the same thing. Flora, microflora, and microbiome are also all the same things. When we are talking about microbes that live in the large intestine, I generally refer to them as gut bugs, intestinal microflora, microbiome, or gut flora. I hope there is no confusion. Bacteria and fungi are not the same thing. Yeast is a type of fungi. Most people still think of yeast as a bad actor on the gut scene, but this is not the case.

Your gut flora's primary job is to extract calories and energy from food items that our bodies are unable to digest. Examples of this are plant fiber, resistant starch, and those parts of foods that are not fully digested in the small intestine. The main action of gut bugs is to turn these undigested foods into fats, vitamins, hormones, and antibiotic-like chemicals for their own self-protection.

As mentioned previously, there are about 100 trillion microorganisms in the intestines. They mostly fall under eight main phyla, but there are also viruses, yeasts, molds, and parasites. Not all of the gut bugs have been identified because of the difficulty in doing so, but every day we learn more. One thing is for certain: a well-functioning gut flora is one that is highly diverse in phyla, genera, and species, and is low in pathogens. When properly cared for and fed, your gut bugs will take care of you for a long time.

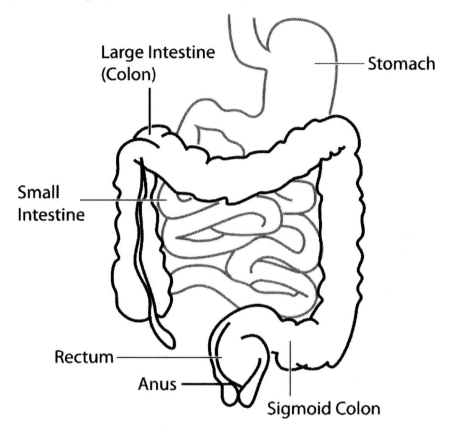

We are a SUPERORGANISM

Another way our relationship with our gut bugs has been described is that of a "Superorganism." This term implies that we (a human host and its trillions of gut bugs) behave as one. We rely on each other and must cooperate to thrive. It also means that sometimes we do things we are compelled to do—like eating, drinking, or seeking out missing nutrients. We coevolved with our gut microbiome, we provide a unique environment for them and in return they give us the tools and chemicals we need to be truly human.

Examples of the superorganisms' powers are the fermentation of indigestible fiber by our gut microbes to produce short chain fatty acids, transformation of bile acids, creation of vitamins, degradation of dietary toxins, the education of the immune system, and the removal of heavy metals from our bloodstream. Acting as a "superorganism," we can get energy and nutrition from foods that would otherwise provide none and we make chemicals not found in nature. The superorganism acts as one, but each part plays an important individual role. Our role in all this is to seek out the proper food sources and avoid extremely toxic situations.

If you remember from earlier, I said the human intestines are populated with approximately 100 trillion gut bugs. All these microbes working together and working for us are often considered a separate organ—just as important to us as a healthy heart or liver. It pays to know what makes your gut bugs tick so that you can treat them right. It wasn't until the 1990's that the full impact of the gut began to be appreciated. So don't feel bad if you are just now hearing of this. With modern equipment and scientists motivated to make new discoveries, more and more amazing benefits of a healthy gut are coming to light every day.

In just the last couple of years, an undeniable connection to diseases like diabetes, rheumatoid arthritis, muscular dystrophy, multiple sclerosis, fibromyalgia, and even some cancers has been established. Obesity might also be caused by an improper mix of microbes in the gut.

Origination of the intestinal microbiome

It seems like almost everybody has an 'a-ha moment' when they come to the realization that our guts become populated with a flourishing community of gut bugs *before birth*. When a baby is still in the womb, its gut was long believed to be sterile. But somehow nature ensured that the first seeds of the future gut biome begin to develop before the baby takes its first breath. As soon as it sucks in those first oxygen molecules, more microbes begin to colonize the baby. These microbes can come from anywhere—the mother's birth canal, the doctor's hands, the air, or other babies nearby.

But, you see, babies are special. They don't have great immune systems and they can't fend for themselves. They rely on their mother for everything—including a healthy gut. Shortly before a baby is born, the soon-to-be mother's gut biome begin to change and rearrange. Often these changes lead to undesirable consequences like rapid weight gain, mood disorders, and (gestational) diabetes—but this is all part of the gut bugs' master plan. They need to prepare the mother to take care of her newborn in ways that she can't on her own.

Bacteria from the mother's gut travel through mysterious channels, known as the enteromammary pathway. Not just any gut bugs, but the ones that the baby needs to keep its gut free of disease. These stimulate the baby's immune system and are meant to keep it healthy for life. Once these bacteria are established inside the mammary glands, the table is set for baby's first meal.

In 2012, Spanish researchers found that "the breast milk received from the mother is one of the factors determining how the bacterial flora will develop in the newborn baby." It was long-thought that breast milk was sterile. With new testing methods, scientists have been very surprised. The latest DNA sequencing methods have proven that there are over 700 different species of microbes living inside of the human breast and are secreted in milk.

Also found in human breast milk, which is often cited as being "fiber free," are hundreds of different fiber types. In fact, a very large percentage of the calories in human breast milk are meant for the bacteria and only indirectly for the baby. This special fiber, known as "Human Milk Oligosaccharide (HMO)," is there for one main purpose—to feed the microbes that are in the baby's gut. The microbes eat this fiber and produce all sorts of chemicals and compounds the baby needs to thrive. But as always, there's more to the story than that.

Milk and Marmalade

By the time a baby is a week or two old, its large intestine should be filled with a certain bacteria called bifidobacteria. Bifidobacteria is a gem of a bacterium in that it can prevent diarrhea, allergies, intestinal bloating and colic in babies. Throughout childhood, bifido walks hand-in-hand with us. It creates an exclusive environment not suitable for pathogenic bacteria. As we transition from milk to marmalade, bifidobacteria is replaced by microbes that enjoy a more varied diet. Also, remember all the HMOs we talked about—they also play a dual role. Pathogenic bacteria LOVE HMOs. As soon as a pathogenic bacterium sees an HMO, it will jump on it. This is an evolutionary 'trick' that is played on bad gut bugs. The HMOs are structurally similar to cell coatings that make them look like an empty piece of intestinal real-estate. Pathogens become attached and try to colonize them. This 'trick,' known as "ligand mimicry," is the primary way that the baby stays healthy and disease free in its first few months of life. Without this, these pathogenic bacteria would instead set up shop in the baby's stomach and small intestine leading to illness. Furthermore, not all of these HMOs are digested by the baby or its gut bugs—some are absorbed into the blood and urine where they further scrub the baby of unwanted pathogens. Remember this idea—it will become important again for the adult.

C-Sections and the Microbiota

It seems that nature put lots of effort into ensuring a baby would end up with a gut filled with a specific type of bacteria, and have plenty to eat for itself and the gut microbes. What happens when a baby is born by Cesarean section and/or not breast fed as is so common nowadays?

Several factors can influence the state of the baby's health. The milk from overweight mothers contains less diversity of microbial species. The type of labor also affects the microbes in the breast milk—mothers who underwent planned C-section show much less microbial diversity in breast milk than those who had emergency C-sections, presumably a connection between the stress of natural childbirth and hormonal signals. Also, the baby itself is colonized by a completely different set of microbes when its entry into the world is not through the birth canal. In babies born naturally, gut microbes are stable within one month. For those delivered through C-section, it can take up to six months for gut flora to stabilize. And finally, formula fed babies show gut bugs completely different from breast fed babies. As is said of breastfeeding over formula feeding:

- It contains active infection-fighting white blood cells and natural chemicals that give increased protection against infections in the first months, when these can be the most serious.
- It can help prevent SIDS, sudden infant death syndrome, according to the American Academy of Pediatrics.
- It contains the perfect proportion of nutrients that your baby needs, including protein, carbohydrates, fat, and calcium.
- It is easily digestible.
- It may protect against allergies and asthma in the future.
- It may decrease a baby's risk of obesity in the future.

- It may contain some fatty acids that promote brain development.
- Breastfeeding can help new mothers lose weight more easily.

Serotonin

Serotonin, or 5-hydroxytryptamine (5-HT), is a monoamine neurotransmitter biochemically derived from tryptophan. Serotonin is responsible for mood, sleep, appetite, memory and learning. 90% of the serotonin in a human is produced in the gut and its effects extend well outside of brain functions.

Serotonin is responsible for gut motility, blood clotting, and as a vasoconstrictor. Serotonin receptors are located throughout the body and once attached to a receptor, serotonin controls the release of other neurotransmitters such as GABA, glutamate, acetylcholine, dopamine, norepinephrine and epinephrine as well as hormones such as cortisol, vasopressin, oxytocin, and prolactin and insulin-like growth factor. Antidepressant medications often act on these same receptors.

If the food you eat contains irritants to the intestine, serotonin is released to make the gut move faster and in some cases causes diarrhea and vomiting. The serotonin receptor responsible for vomiting is known as 5HT3 and is a target for controlling nausea caused by chemotherapy.

Scientists from University College Cork discovered that when gut bacteria were absent in early life, brain disorders related to a lack of serotonin were seen in later life and that a correction of these gut bacteria did not reverse the damage. This is an obvious case of the gut influencing the development of the brain and should give anyone pause before administering antibiotics to a child.

Microbes as we Mature

The maturation of gut microbes into an adult-like configuration happens during the first three years of life. There are no gut bugs unique to babies or adults, but there are unique patterns. These patterns shift as we grow, travel, and eat different foods. The establishment of your intestinal microbiota is a progressive process. This process of increasing diversity is required for healthy growth and is important for nearly every aspect of your life. By the end of a human's second year, we see the gut bugs begin to progress through a cycle which has been described as:

- Nutrient absorption and food fermentation
- Stimulation of the host immune system
- Barrier effects against pathogens

As one approaches their teenage years, this process is complete, and the ecosystem displays extreme stability in healthy adults. In the days of yore, people ate real food and did things people are supposed to do: They lifted heavy objects, slept according to the sun, ate when hungry, ingested microbes, and often went without food. Recent studies show that the biggest dangers to upsetting the intestinal microbiome are:

- Environment
- Diet
- Stress
- Antibiotics
- Age
- Season

Each one of these can be mitigated to some extent if you know a few tricks.

When properly cared for, our gut bugs should provide us a long, healthy life. However, as we age, changes to the composition of our gut microbes begin to occur and can have detrimental effects on the elderly. Our bodies age. There is nothing we can do about it. One thing we can do; is control *how* we age.

It has recently been discovered that the changing microbial structure in the gut of the elderly causes a reduction in the gut's immune system, or the Gastro-associated Lymphoid Tissue. Alterations of the GALT make one more susceptible to infection—an extremely troubling concern for the elderly especially in an assisted-living situation. A reduction in the GALT allows for uncontrolled microbial growth with no way to stop the pathogens from taking over from the beneficial microbes. Here you see great battles being fought, only without the normal weapons—mucus, defensins, and antimicrobial peptides which have all been significantly reduced in old age.

At this point, it's easy to enter a "death spiral," these weakened defenses cause localized inflammation, inflammation favors a bloom of pathological bacteria and viruses, repeated attacks by pathogens cause system wide inflammation. This unfortunate combination of events has been termed "inflamm-ageing."

It has been recently hypothesized that from an evolutionary perspective, our human microbiome is performing a "clock like function" in the human ageing process. By providing us with metabolic and defense functions, intestinal microbes can improve human fitness in the early life, but, through a twist of evolutionary fate, may also try to remove unhealthy individuals in old age in order to free resources for younger members of the population—life can be cruel.

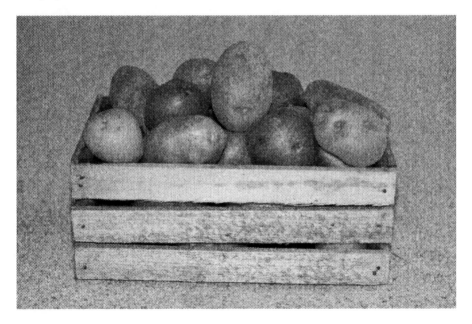

While this may seem a harsh reality, it is a matter of fact that as we age and our other systems begin to disintegrate, so does our gut microbiome. If this all occurs at an extraordinarily advanced age, it's considered normal. But in our modern society, this is being seen at younger and younger ages and people in their 30s and 40s are exhibiting illnesses that were previously only seen in those of advanced age.

As the body itself does not all age at the exact same rate, neither does the gut microbiome. Science is just now beginning to understand the importance of gut function on aging. When the gut and its microbial inhabitants are viewed as separate organs, we can begin to control not "whether" one ages, but "how" one ages. Diet, stress, sleep, and environmental factors are easily manipulated. If simple changes can have profound effects on gut microbes, age-related illnesses may be reserved for the truly elderly and people will live their final years in relative good health.

The Brain-Gut Connection

As some of the microbes in our gut can produce brain chemicals (neurotransmitters), schizophrenia, depression, bipolar disorder and other neurochemical imbalances have been positively connected to a poor gut microbiome. The undeniable interactions between our intestinal microbiome and our gray matter has been termed the "brain-gut connection." It's long been known that the brain can exert control over the stomach: Butterflies in your stomach at the thought of public speaking, a knot in your stomach when you witness a horrific crime, and scientists discovered that digestive processes begin at the mere thought of eating delicious food.

However, it's only recently been discovered that the brain-gut connection is actually a two-way street. In a recent edition of the *Scientific American*, the brain-gut connection was beautifully described:

> "Technically known as the enteric nervous system, the second brain consists of sheaths of neurons embedded in the walls of the long tube of our gut, or alimentary canal, which measures about nine meters end to end from the esophagus to the anus. The second brain contains some 100 million neurons, more than in either the spinal cord or the peripheral nervous system. This multitude of neurons in the enteric nervous system enables us to "feel" the inner world of our gut and its contents."

This amazing new discovery of the brain-gut connection should be enough reason for everyone to ensure they have the healthiest guts possible. For millions of years, no one had to give any thought to the brain-gut connection...*it just was*. What has changed? The answer should be obvious. Once upon a time, we were all born with perfect guts that only got better as we scraped and grubbed our way through life. Now, the fairy tale is gone. If we happen to be born with a great array of gut bugs, they go downhill with the first round of baby-antibiotics we get and when are weaned off our gut-bug friendly milk, we eat junk food. It's modern life that's taking its toll.

Factor S

One of the biggest factors in our overall health is sleep. Deprive yourself of it and your health deteriorates rapidly. One convincing demonstration of the Brain-Gut Connection is a molecule secreted by gut bugs known as "Factor S." One phase of our sleep-cycle is known as slow-wave sleep. This cycle is known as "deep sleep" and is the time when the brain recovers from its daily activities and new thoughts are 'cut and pasted' into the long-term memory drives of your brain. This is also when human growth hormone is secreted and dreams are formed. Disruptions in this cycle can result in bedwetting, nightmares, and sleep-walking. In other words—it's a very important part of our 40 winks.

Gut bugs have a massive hand in ensuring we get a good night's sleep, and in turn, our entire physiology. They want us to remember where that wonderful patch of microbe-encrusted wild onions is and they want us to have the strength to get there again. Factor S is how they do it. As animals get sleepy, Factor S accumulates in their brain and promotes sleep onset and the shift into slow-wave sleep. Additionally, other brain chemicals such as the well – known serotonin and melatonin are generated by gut bugs and contribute further to our vivid dreams, rest and recuperation.

GABA

Researchers at Baylor College of Medicine and Texas Children's Hospital have identified commensal bacteria in the human intestine that produce a neurotransmitter that may play a role in preventing or treating inflammatory bowel diseases such as Crohn's disease.

γ-Aminobutyric acid; or GABA, is the chief inhibitory neurotransmitter in the mammalian central nervous system where it plays a role in regulating neuronal excitability. In humans, GABA is also directly responsible for the regulation of muscle tone. The Baylor researchers identified a strain of bacteria, Bifidobacterium dentium, that secretes large amounts of GABA.

One of GABAs interesting side-effects is the lowering of inflammation. Immune cells in the gut have GABA receptors and when these receptors were activated, inflammatory factors decreased, leading the researchers to believe that Bifidobacterium dentium could be targeted to reduce the inflammation associated with inflammatory bowel diseases.

Immunity

The immune system keeps us alive by recognizing and destroying harmful microbes while leaving beneficial ones alone. As soon as a baby is born, bacteria, fungi, and even viruses begin to colonize its entire body. The very first microbes that reach the baby's immune centers set the stage for lifelong immunity.

Most of our immune system lies within the gut. This makes perfect sense since our gut interacts with the outside environment—food and water. The gut-associated lymphoid tissue consists of specialized immune cells, known as Peyer's Patches, and it's one of the largest immune system organs in humans, containing up to 70% of the body's immune tissues. Peyer's Patches contain specialized receptors known as B and T cells that recognize and disable pathogens and viruses.

In easier to understand terms, these Peyer's Patches which are found throughout the intestines, are 'smart' devices which can 'learn' to recognize harmful microbes and viruses. When you get an immunization, it's the Peyer's Patches which sense the injected virus and build up an immunity for it should you encounter the virus again.

Inside Out

The *insides* of the intestines are *outside* of the body.

Think about that for a moment. Just like your skin, the intestines are subject to an onslaught of outside influences—but unlike your skin, your intestines must be able to absorb minerals, vitamins, and energy from food. The only way it can do this is to kill anything it doesn't want to get *into* the body.

The conventional wisdom view of the immune system, and the immune system taught in medical school, is that of a complex assembly of organs, tissues, cells, and chemicals that eliminate pathogens. A newer view needs to include the fact that our immune system has evolved to control microbes and that microbes control the immune system. When the immune system is not in tip-top working condition, it causes a chain reaction of events leading to autoimmune conditions and inflammatory diseases such as multiple sclerosis, psoriasis, juvenile diabetes, rheumatoid arthritis, Crohn's disease, and autoimmune uveitis. The quicker mainstream medical establishments recognize the power of microbes and diet on the parts of the immune system that lie in the gut, the quicker we will eliminate many diseases.

The immune system with its Peyer's Patches, T and B cells are a front-line defense, but they need lots of fuel. Earlier I mentioned a key role of gut bugs is to produce short chain fatty acids (SCFA), well, guess what fuels the immune system...SCFA. This special fat turns untrained T cells into powerful T regulator cells and strengthens the entire gut lining. The surest way to get plenty of SCFA and fuel for your immune "machine" is to eat plenty of fiber—particularly resistant starch as found in the potato hack in large amounts.

Preventing allergy

Closely related to the immune system is the ability of gut microbes to prevent allergies. Allergies are simply an overreaction of the immune system to non-harmful substances.

Gut bugs are amazing creatures, have I mentioned that? They have developed what is known as toll-like receptors on their exteriors that recognize anything that isn't friendly. Once this identification is made, they spring into action and call for help. This help can be in the form of destroying invading pathogens or repairing damage done by poisons or even by radiation.

Gut bugs can also initiate a sequence known as "oral tolerance". Oral tolerance is first seen when babies put everything in their mouth, the gut bugs sense these different 'germs' and store them in their databanks for future reference. In this manner, the immune system is trained by the baby to react when it later encounters these substances. Oral tolerance can also be used later in life to train the immune system to react to specific pathogens. Minute traces of a known pathogen are placed in the mouth and through mysterious pathways, gut bugs identify and protect against that pathogen. When this system is broken, as with a gut populated by pathogenic bacteria and with widespread inflammation, the remaining microbes overreact to everything in a last-ditch attempt to protect its host. This causes allergies to escalate at an alarming rate.

Repression of pathogenic microbial growth

The intestinal microflora, as a whole, performs a function called "the barrier effect." This is its way of keeping unwanted microbes, viruses, and other harmful growths out of the intestines. The barrier effect is also known as competitive exclusion, and relies on a healthy, vigorous growth of beneficial microbes to "crowd out" any harmful ones—it's one of the more elegantly simple mechanisms of the gut microbiome and one that is employed by creatures big and small throughout the world, even humans do it with their exclusive membership clubs, jobs, and the "good ol' boy" networks commonly seen.

This barrier effect protects us from both invading species and species already inside us that are only helpful in small populations. Many of our friendly bacteria rely in other friendlies for their food—in this sense, these microbes are helpful to us and to each other. It's these tight knit bonds that especially strengthen the barrier effect and invading species that are out only for themselves cannot get in.

The barrier effect is made even stronger by bacteria and fungi who possess special weapons, known as defensins and bacteriocins. Some gut bugs produce numerous short chain fatty acids which lower the pH in the intestines, this makes for an inhospitable breeding ground for pathogens.

This barrier effect is only as good as the human host makes it—starve your gut bugs of their preferred foods, kill them off with antibiotics, or live a life of high stress and you've essentially ruined the barrier effect. Conversely, a diet high in foods the gut bugs thrive on like resistant starch, plant fibers, and low in foods they don't like will provide a nearly impenetrable gut.

In the end...

The human gut has been the subject of fascination since man developed a wondering mind. Unfortunately, we know more about our solar system than we do the 20-some feet of tube that stretches from our mouth to our rectum. Only recently have the inhabitants of our intestinal microbiome been thought of beyond the disease and discomforts of such denizens as E. coli and Salmonella. Now, we are not only picking and choosing which microbes we desire but we are learning to build perfect guts and we've started to learn their names. The information explosion of the last few decades has not been lost on our guts—we are compiling data from around the world and scientists are feverishly trying to catalog and categorize the genes that make up 90% of us so that we may thrive as a species. If the trend of the last hundred years to destroy our guts with antibiotics and pretend that gut bugs "just are" isn't completely reversed, then we might as well bid adieu to any hope that our children's children will have much of a chance at a long, healthy life.

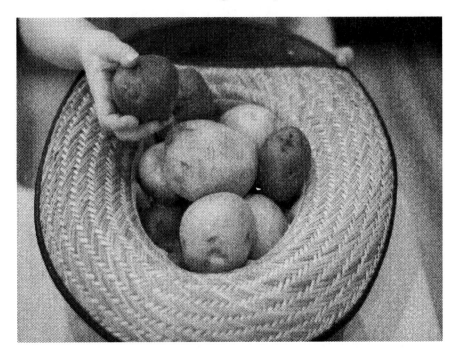

It's not important for everyone to have a thorough understanding of the intricacies of their gut any more than you need to know what makes your car go. But when your "check engine" light comes on, you'd better know what to do! The human species "check engine" light has been on for centuries—and our warranty is expired. Don't leave it up to science, the medical profession, or Dr. Oz to tell you what to do...you're in the middle of the desert and there's no tow-truck coming. Buzzards are circling. The next move is yours.

Final Thoughts

If the potato hack does not sit so well on your stomach and you are not feeling the "potato love," it could simply be because your gut inhabitants are not used to digesting potatoes. As most people in the world eat several pounds of potatoes per week, the potatoes are well-suited for most people.

If the potato hack treats you well, ie. you lose weight and feel great, consider making these starchy tubers a big part of your life. But don't just stop there, introduce your gut to all the starchy gut food found in nature: rice, beans, green bananas, etc… and maybe even a spoonful or two of my favorite white powder, potato starch.

POTATO QUOTES

"YOU SHOULD GET DOWN ON YOUR HANDS AND KNEES AND PRAISE THE POTATO!"

DR. JOHN MCDOUGALL (VIA YOUTUBE)

Notes:

Chapter 12. FAQs

You'd be surprised how many questions the potato hack generates. While I'd like to think I've answered all of the possible questions you could have; I know that there will still be questions. I love when people ask questions. I love asking questions. In class, I'm always the annoying person with his hand up asking things. Please have a look at these frequently asked questions and if you still need answers, hop on over to my blog at www.potatohack.com and ask away.

I'll divide these FAQs into three sections:

• Potato Hack Questions
• Resistant Starch Questions
• General Health Questions

Potato Hack FAQs:

Can't I just use [insert food item here] instead of potatoes?

Answer — Maybe. I have only researched the use of white potatoes. Sweet potatoes and yams seem the most likely substitute. I doubt most foods, especially meats or green veggies would work very well. You could probably lose some weight eating any single food for a few days, but the magic of the potato hack is in the potato itself. The potato contains a special combination of chemicals that make it ideal for long term weight loss and short term fat burning. Lots of science in the science chapter on this.

Can I also eat [insert food item here]?

Answer — The added meat variation allows a bit of meat on potato hack days, but if you want results, stick to potatoes when eating. The simplicity of the potato hack is part of its magic. If you are eating something that is not a potato, you are doing it all wrong.

Do I need to peel the potatoes?

Answer – Case-by-case. If the potato has green spots or eyes, peel it. If it's from a big supermarket chain and not labeled organic, peel it. Otherwise, enjoy the peels, they have lots of fiber.

Are organic potatoes worth the extra money?

Answer – I think so. I have a degree in biotechnology, I am not at all a fan of GMO foods, though most in this field don't think that way. Soon it will be impossible to tell if a food is GMO or not, unless specifically labeled "organic." Besides GMO issues, organic produce should not have the chemicals conventional potatoes have on them from pesticides, herbicides, and fungicides. Organic potatoes are not that much more expensive.

Why do snorers stop snoring on the potato hack?

Answer – I'm convinced it has to do with a very strong anti-inflammatory action. There is a lot of tissue in the throat (ie. lymph glands, tonsils, adenoids, salivary glands) that are subject to inflammation. A slight reduction can be enough to allow a habitual snorer to get a good night's sleep.

What's your favorite recipe?

Answer – Oil-less hashbrowns

What's your favorite variation?

Answer – Potatoes by Day (PBD)

What's the deal with blue/purple potatoes?

Answer – Cool, eh? They stay blue even after being cooked, so they make a really fun addition to potato salad, especially on the 4th of July. The antioxidants that make them blue are shown to have some extraordinary cancer fighting effects. They taste just like regular potatoes and grow well anywhere potatoes are grown.

Must I cook and cool potatoes on the potato hack?

Answer – Nope, but it's wise to do a batch so you have them on hand for snacking "emergencies." If you are worried about RS, don't worry. The potato hack is a high RS diet no matter what.

Won't all the carbs make me fat?

Answer — Nope! Most unintentional weight gain is caused by over eating and insulin resistance. The potato hack helps both.

Won't I lose muscle?

Answer — Not in 3-5 days you won't. Your body likes its muscles, it will keep them as long as it can. Since you are not starving, your body will spare your muscles and fuel with fat. Potatoes are a great protein source, anyway.

Can I try exercising/weight lifting while potato hacking?

Answer — Sure, try all you like. But why? Take a break, you probably need it.

How long can I safely do the potato hack?

Answer — Chris Voigt set the bar with 60 days. I like to recommend 3-5 days at a stretch but have done 14 days. Two weeks is the most I would advise, there are some nutritional deficiencies involved, so get replenished and start again. It won't set you back.

How does the potato hack affect a ketogenic diet?

Answer — Hard to say. It depends on the amount of insulin resistance you developed while eating a keto diet. The potato hack itself often proves ketogenic as your body is burning so much body fat. Seems crazy, but can be easily tested with Ketostix.

How does the potato hack affect my gut microbes?

Answer — Gut microbes love the potato hack. In fact, if there is one aspect of the potato diet that outshines the rest, it's the impact it has on gut bacteria. When fed a continual supply of RS rich potatoes, your gut bacteria are allowed to grow and evolve, creating a diverse ecosystem that's often missing when eating a Western diet with its ever-changing food-scape. See my gut results and discussion.

Why are potatoes banned on the Paleo® diet?

Answer — Stupidity? The "official" reason is because potatoes were not available to our distant ancestors, so we should not eat them, either. But yams were, and they are also banned. The "unofficial" reason is simply because they contain too many carbs, and Paleo® is simply a low carb diet. Word has it they are slowly coming around.

Can I do the potato hack while pregnant or nursing?

Answer — I would advise against it while pregnant, but just because it may put you in too much of an overall calorie deficit to "eat for two." Potato hacking while breast feeding should be perfectly fine. However, I do not recommend potato hacking while nursing a baby as this may put unneeded stress on you.

Can a diabetic do the potato hack?

Answer — With caution. If you go into this knowing you have glucose control issues, please take some time to ascertain what the potato hack is doing to your blood sugar. Pre-diabetics on no meds may find the potato hack returns them to normal. Well-controlled T2Ds may find they need less meds. T1Ds will always need their therapeutic insulin and should check BG continually as a precaution.

In 10 words or less, convince me to try the potato hack.

Answer — It's simple, cheap, and you won't be hungry.

What do the following acronyms stand for: CICO, SAD, PH, FBG, PP, BG, RS

Answer — Calories in, calories out; standard American diet; potato hack; fasting blood glucose; postprandial; blood glucose; resistant starch

Resistant Starch FAQs:

What are RS1, 2, 3 and 4?

Answer – Different types of resistant starch.

Which is the best RS?

Answer – There is no "best" only different. All types of RS have proven effective in human studies for increasing gut health.

Isn't RS just fiber?

Answer – Yes, but it's specifically fermentable fiber that preferentially feeds beneficial gut bacteria.

I read *Fiber Menace*, isn't fiber bad for us?

Answer – No. <u>Fiber Menace</u> was written years before the science on the importance of gut health. Gut bacteria used to be treated as a "bad" thing, now we know how crucial it is to human health and that bacteria need fiber to thrive.

Do I still need to supplement with RS on the potato hack?

Answer – No. The potato hack is high in RS no matter how you do it. But you can if you like.

Why do you like potato starch so much?

Answer – Because I can make it at home. It's one of the few supplements that the supplement industry has not commercialized…yet.

What is persorption?

Answer – Starch granules have been shown to get absorbed [technically "persorbed"] through the gastrointestinal tract and enter blood circulation. There are a few speculative papers that show this could lead to harm. However, every single starchy meal you eat causes persorption of starch granules. If it were dangerous, I think we'd know by now. There may also be a positive side to persorption. Pathogenic bacteria cling to the starch granules. Starch granules in the blood may help eliminate pathogens from the body.

How much RS or fiber should we eat in a day?

Answer – Shoot for 30-50g of fiber per day from real food. If you fall short, supplement with potato starch, inulin, or the fiber of your choice.

Where can I find a good list of RS contents in foods?

Answer – There are none. Potatoes, green bananas, beans, corn, wheat, and rice are good sources, but the levels change with ripeness and cooking methods, so exact amounts need to be determined in a lab for each food.

Why does RS make me fart?

Answer – Farting is a byproduct of bacterial fermentation. This means that the bacteria in your large intestine are feeding on the RS and producing gas. They also produce a host of other compounds, such as butyrate.

General Health FAQs:

How do I determine if my gut is healthy?

Answer — By how you feel. If you have continual "modern, dyspeptic gut" symptoms, frequent noxious farts, or experience diarrhea and constipation on a regular basis your gut is unhealthy. If you poop daily, rarely have indigestion or heartburn, and can eat just about anything then you have a healthy gut. Fixing an unhealthy gut may be a lifelong endeavor for some. For others, a shift in diet may be all it takes.

Are there any specific gut bacteria we need?

Answer — Yes, but by eating a plant-heavy diet you will get all of the right bacteria. The science is too young to accurately tell you which bacteria you are missing.

What are SIBO, IBS, IBD, and leaky gut?

Answer — Small Intestinal Bacterial Overgrowth, Irritable Bowel Syndrome, Inflammatory Bowel Disease. These are all gut problems that can possibly be helped with RS and the potato hack.

What is the difference between prebiotics and probiotics?

Answer — Probiotics are helpful bacteria used to supplement your own bacteria, ie. Bifidobacteria. Prebiotics are food for the bacteria already present in your gut and thought to stimulate mainly the beneficial bacteria while starving out the pathogens.

What is the best diet plan to follow?

Answer — One that you thrive on. One that contains ample plant matter. One that does not discriminate against any real, whole food. One that shuns modern, processed foods.

The "No Guru Zone"

Before you start to think I have all the answers, I want to clear something up. I am not a guru—I'm just a guy whose been talking about all this for 5-years. Every great diet out there has its associated "guru's." There's Loren Cordain of the Paleo Diet®, Dr. Atkins of the Atkin's Diet®. Dr. Agatston invented the South Beach Diet®, and Jenny Craig, well, you know get the drift...

Trademarked diets are big money-makers. Not only do they spawn books, television shows, and videos, but they also create a need for numerous products. Trademarked diets and their cult-like leaders become industries. I hate gurus. I hate the way diets become religions. I hate that people stick to diets because they are so invested, financially and emotionally, yet they are seeing no benefits. Battle lines get drawn between vegans and meat-eaters. Low carb vs high carb. It makes no sense! We are all different, and what we fail to see is that we are getting sucked into these diets by slick marketing and persuasive leaders. One needs only to look at Subway's Jared Fogle to see what guru status does to a person.

The potato hack is a "no guru zone." I like talking about the potato hack, but it will never be an industry...there's just no money in it. In fact, the potato hack is the exact opposite of all other diets out there. Everyone who tries it, and likes it, becomes an instant guru. The potato hack is customizable, there are hundreds of possible combinations. I have no doubt that someone will come along and try to capitalize on the potato diet, selling the "perfect" potatoes at double the normal cost, selling secret herbs that will make the potato hack more effective, or devising some method of ensuring that the money you save on the potato hack ends up in their pocket.

I suspect Big Diet would love to discredit the potato hack. I have no doubt that soon there will be those that claim this is all a hoax or that it is somehow dangerous. This entire book is mainly designed to give you freedom from the diet industry. A poke in the eye to Big Diet and its gurus. I've done my best to show you what was discovered in 1849 is still valid today and that the simple potato holds great promise to setting us free from the tyranny of the great powers that are, in fact, keeping us dependent on trademarked diets.

The only thing I'll insist you buy is *potatoes.*

POTATO QUOTES

"ONLY TWO THINGS IN THIS WORLD ARE TOO SERIOUS TO BE JESTED ON, POTATOES AND MATRIMONY."

— OLD IRISH SAYING

Notes:

APPENDIX A. POTATO HISTORY

Much of the magic of potatoes involves the symbiotic relationship between humans and starchy foods. Even though the *first* hominids did not have access to potatoes, they did have access to starchy tubers. Indeed, since before man walked on two legs, he was eating starch. Until man migrated out of Africa, he ate yams, roots, seeds and other starchy foods we wouldn't recognize today. As man wandered north into the colder climates of Europe, he found cattails and their starchy roots as well as oats, wheat, and other starchy grains. Those that wandered to the East discovered other suitable replacements for the starches they evolved on. In Asia, they found all kinds of tubers, gourds, and roots, but relied heavily on the starchy sago, which they harvested from the insides of sago palm trees.

In the frozen north along the Bering Land Bridge, they dined on Eskimo potatoes (*Hedysarum alpinum*) and seeds of grasses growing on glacial moraine. As man wandered south into North America, he encountered all kinds of new starch sources like beans and squash. In Northern Mexico, we found corn. Seven thousand years ago, man settled in the lush valleys and high mountains of the Andes mountain range along the west coast of South America—here they discovered potatoes.

High on the windswept, rocky hillsides, man encountered an unlikely food source. Found at elevations as high as 15,000 feet, the early settlers of the Andes were impressed by the vigor and storage qualities of the potato. They found they could thrive on potatoes for most of the year when other foods were scarce. For over 6,000 years, civilizations flourished in the region with the help of the potato.

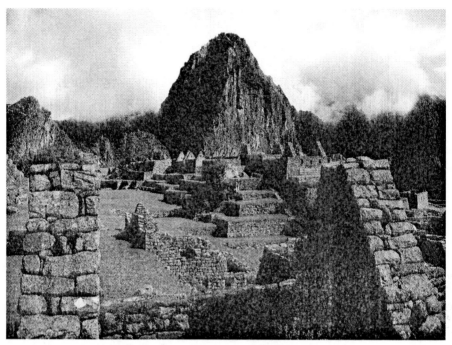

Machu Pichu, Peru, Inca, Andes (Pixabay.com)

In his book, *1493*, Charles Mann described how potatoes were used by the Andean Incans:

> *Potatoes would not seem obvious candidates for domestication. Wild tubers are laced with solanine and tomatine, toxic compounds thought to defend the plants against attacks from dangerous organisms like fungi, bacteria, and human beings. Cooking often breaks down a plant's chemical defenses – many beans for example are safe to eat only after being soaked and heated – but solanine and tomatine are unaffected by the pot and oven. Andean people apparently neutralized them by eating dirt: clay to be precise. In the altiplano, guanacos and vicunas (wild relatives of the llama) lick clay before eating poisonous plants. The toxins in the floage stick – more technically absorb – to the fine clay particles. Bound to dirt the harmful substances pass through the animals' digestive system without affecting it. Mimick-*

ing this process, Indians apparently dunked wild potatoes in a "gravy" made of clay and water. Eventually they bred less lethal varieties, though some of the old poisonous varieties still remain, favored for their resistance to frost. Bags of clay dust are still sold in mountain markets to accompany them on the table. (Charles Mann, 2011)

Humankind definitely benefitted from the discovery of potatoes. By the time Europeans arrived in the Andes thousands of years later, they found the locals eating potatoes in every conceivable way:

Andean Indians ate potatoes boiled, baked and mashed as people in Europe and North America do. But they also consumed them in forms still little known outside the highlands. Potatoes were boiled, peeled, chopped and dried to make papas secas; fermented for months in stagnant water to create a sticky, odoriferous toqosh; ground to pulp, soaked in a jug, and filtered to produce almidón de papa (potato starch). The most ubiquitous concoction was chuno, made by spreading potatoes outside to freeze on cold nights. As it expands the ice inside potato cell walls ruptures cell walls. The potatoes are thawed by morning sun, then frozen again the next night. Repeated freeze-thaw cycles transform the spuds into soft, juicy blobs. Farmers squeeze out the water and produce chuno: stiff styrofoam like nodules about two-thirds smaller than the original tubers. Long exposure to the sun turns them gray-black; cooked into a spicy Andean stew, they resemble gnocchi, the potato-flour dumplings favored in central Italy. Chuno can be kept for years without refrigeration, meaning that it can be stored as insurance against bad harvests. It was the food that sustained the conquering Inca armies. (Charles Mann, 1493)

Many of these traditional potato dishes are available on Amazon and other marketplaces:

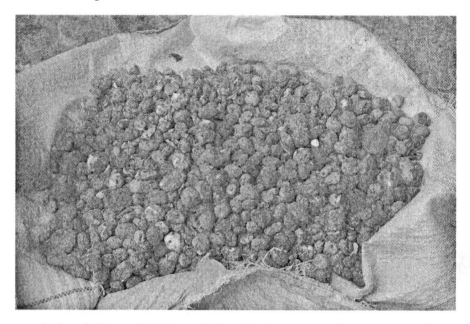

"Chuno" (Freeze-dried Potatoes) Photo Credit: Eric in SF [CC BY-SA 3.0]

When the first Spanish Conquistadors arrived in South America, they were most impressed with the potato. In 1570, the first potato made its way to Europe and changed the course of history.

Introduced to Europeans

Though the potato was prolific and hardy, the Spanish put it to very limited use as food for the "underclasses" and to feed hospital patients and prison inmates. It would take 30 more years for the potato to spread to the rest of Europe. In 1780 the people of Ireland adopted the potato for its ability to produce abundant, nutritious food. Unlike any other major crop, potatoes contain most of the vitamins needed for sustenance. Perhaps more importantly, potatoes could provide enough sustenance to feed nearly 10 people on an acre of land. This was the prime factor which caused a population explosion in the early 1800s. Of course, by the mid-1800s the Irish would become so dependent upon this crop that its failure would provoke a famine.

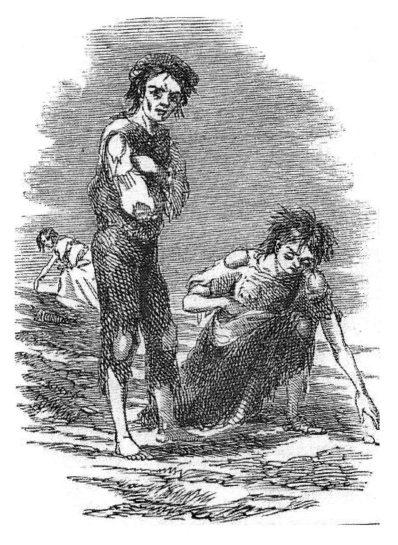

"The scene at Skibbereen, west Cork, in 1847." From a series of illustrations by Cork artist James Mahony (1810-1879), commissioned by Illustrated London News 1847.
(Public Domain)

In France the potato was imposed upon society by Antoine Augustine Parmentier [a *Potato Hack* icon!]. This intellectual saw that the nutritional benefits of the crop combined with its productive capacity could be a boon to the French farmer. He was a pharmacist, chemist and employee of Louis XV. Parmentier discovered the benefits of the potato while held prisoner by the Prussians during the Seven Years' War. He was so amazed by the potato that he vowed it would become a staple of the French diet.

After failing to convince Frenchmen of its advantages, he took a more circular route to make his point.

According to the history books, Parmentier acquired a miserable and unproductive spot of ground on the outskirts of Paris. There, he planted 50 acres of potatoes. During the day, he set a guard over it. This drew considerable attention in the neighborhood. In the evening the guard was relaxed and the locals came to see what all the fuss was about. Believing this plant must be valuable, many peasants "acquired" some of the potatoes from the plot, and soon were growing the root in their own garden plots. Their resistance was overcome by their curiosity and desire to better their lot with the obviously valuable new produce.

(Re)Introduced to America

Soon the potato made its way back over the Atlantic to North America. As time passed, the potato would become *the* major starch source of the world. But not without a few hiccups. In the 1840s a blight wiped out potato crops throughout Europe, and with it came the destruction and dislocation of many of the populations that had become dependent upon it. The Potato Famine in Ireland cut the Irish population in half!

I doubt many people realize the importance of the potato to the Irish in 1700-1800. Prior to the establishment of potato crops, the vast majority of the population got most of their nutrition from oats. Oats as a food staple were problematic and frequent periods of starvation existed. Potatoes were brought to Ireland around the year 1600. By 1700, it had replaced the acreage devoted previously to oats, and more. Potatoes grew readily in soils that would not support oats or other crops. Many millions of families lived upon one acre farmsteads where they raised a single cow and grew several tons of potatoes. Acre for acre, potatoes were light years ahead of any other food crop the Irish had ever known.

By many accounts, in the late 1700s and early 1800s, about 50% of the Irish population was subsisting on potatoes and a bit of milk from their family cow. Seasonally fish were available, but little other meat was eaten. History records a time of population growth and healthy, hearty people eating potatoes. Numerous surveys showed that the Irish people were eating upwards of 14 pounds of potatoes per day (working men) with less being eaten by women, children, and the elderly. Potatoes were eaten at each of the three daily meals, washed down with milk, water, or whiskey.

The countries sole reliance on potatoes was its downfall. In the 1840s, back-to-back failures of the entire potato crop due to a bacterial disease known as "potato blight" caused widespread malnutrition and death.

The Last 100 Years

Over the past 100 years, the "civilized" world began a new relationship with the potato. Though potatoes are the #4 food crop (behind wheat, corn, and rice), hardly any potatoes are eaten in their whole, fresh form. Potatoes have become the staple of the fast-food industry where French fries take center stage in drive-through meals. Deep-fried potatoes such as French fries, tater tots, and potato chips (crisps) are consumed in much greater quantity than boiled or baked potatoes. Even when consumed fresh, potatoes are more of a delivery vehicle for butter, sour cream, and bacon.

Potatoes can be eaten as part of a healthy diet, but only if we eat them the way nature presents them. Potatoes eaten as they were in the 1840's when they were predominantly baked, roasted, boiled, or steamed are a super-food if there ever was one.

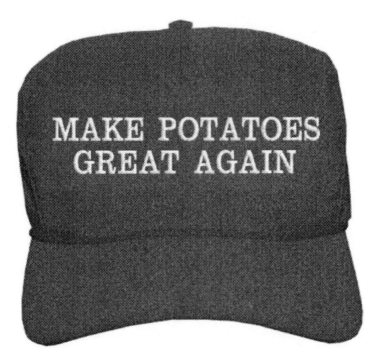

Notes:

APPENDIX B. LET'S GET GROWING!

Potatoes are my favorite garden plant. They have beautiful foliage and flowers, require little care, and give a massive return for the investment. I've been growing potatoes on a large scale for over 10-years on my little homestead in the far north of Alaska. I typically harvest 300-400 pounds of mature potatoes. Picked in late September, these potatoes last in my garage until April. As soon as the snow melts, I plant the potatoes that are left.

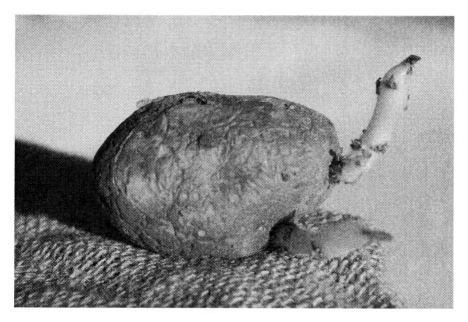

Sprouted Potato (Author's Photo)

Why Plant Potatoes?

Potatoes from the supermarket are an industrial commodity. Unless "organic" they have undoubtedly been treated with many chemicals. In a large growing operation, potatoes are sprayed in the field with pesticides and herbicides. Prior to harvest, some farmers spray them with chemicals that kill the leaves so they are easier to dig. After harvest, potatoes are treated with fungicides and also sprout inhibitors so that they do not begin to grow.

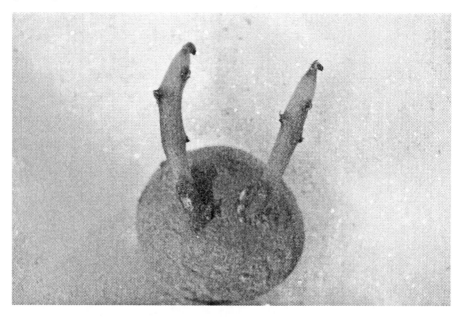

Spike Spud (Author's Photo)

The worst chemical that potatoes are treated with are most likely the sprout inhibitors. One sprout inhibitor, Chlorprophame, is commonly found on store-bought potatoes in levels that exceed the safety limits set by the USDA and FDA. Due to recently discovered health concerns, the EPA has classified Chlorophame as a "carbamate" and has placed strict limits on the amount of residue that can remain on potatoes. Some countries have even banned the use of Chlorophame.

Though long considered non-toxic and safe, this type of sprout inhibitor is actually a carbamate. Carbamates had a short-lived medicinal use but were found to be toxic and ineffective. Carbamates are more commonly found in urethane, used in paint and wood preservatives. As farmers search for better methods of sprout prevention, Chlorophame continues to see widespread use in the US.

In addition to the chemicals, many people are against genetically modified (GMO) plants. There are several GMO potato varieties in test trials and undoubtedly coming to a supermarket near you in the near future.

Should we avoid all supermarket potatoes? No, but please wash and peel them well. Choose organic if possible. Or do as I do…grow your own.

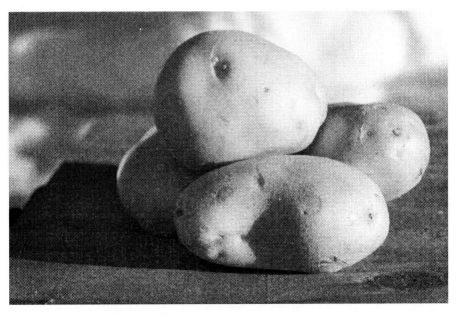

Yukon Gold (Author's Photo)

Potato Growing Tips

If you are an avid gardener, potatoes will be one of the easiest crops you grow. If you were not born with a green thumb, but want to try, you will find easy success following these tips.

Potatoes enjoy sandy, loose soil with a slightly acidic pH of 5.8 to 6.5. Luckily, this describes most garden soil. Potatoes can be grown in any soil type, but for best results, it should be easy to dig and not stay wet. Potatoes do best when planted in rows with about 2-3 feet between rows.

Potatoes are an underground tuber; in case you didn't know. They grow from a potato that has sprouted (called eyes). Potatoes can also be grown from seed, but this method is rarely employed due to the time it takes compared to planting a sprouted potato.

> *In view of the fact that the potato is a pernicious substance whose use can cause leprosy, it is hereby forbidden, under pain of fine, to cultivate it. (French Law, 1763)*

The potatoes grow underground, above the seed potato. To maximize harvest, it's advisable to mound dirt on top of the potatoes as they grow. Commercial farmers know this little trick, too and spend considerable effort to make a suitable place to grow potatoes.

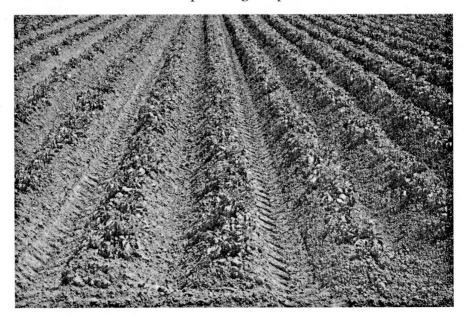

Potato Hills (Pixabay.com)

These mounds can easily be made in a home garden with a shovel, hoe, or roto-tiller attachment. A little bit of work pays huge dividends when it comes to growing a decent crop of spuds. Even if you don't have a garden or a good place to plant a row of potatoes, they are also easily grown in simple containers. Some people just buy a bag of garden soil, make a slit in each one, and plant a potato right in the bag.

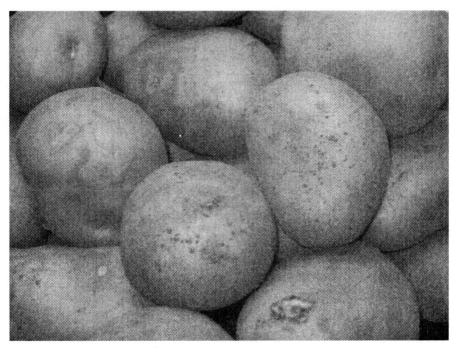

Piles o' Potatoes (Author's Photo)

Buying Seed Potato

Notice I said *"seed* potato" and not "potato *seeds."* You will get a chuckle at the local garden center if you ask for potato seeds. Seed potatoes are small potatoes that were saved from last year's harvest and stored in a cool place all winter. In the spring, they are allowed to sprout and sold as "seed potatoes."

Choose whatever type potato you like. Try a couple different varieties. Most garden centers will have Yukon Gold, Russetts, and some type of red potato. Resist the urge to plant sweet potatoes unless you know they grow in your area. Sweet potatoes are a tropical plant and quite picky about where they grow. Regular "white" potatoes grow pretty much anywhere from the Arctic Circle to the equator.

Seed catalogs are also a great place to buy seed potatoes. Most companies will take your order early and ship at the exact right time for your climate zone.

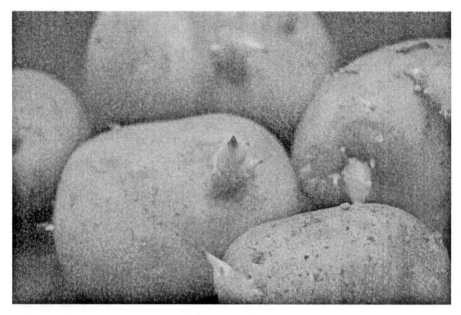

Lovely Eyes (Author's Photo)

Planting

As soon as soil can be worked in the spring, dig a shallow trench in your garden and lay the seed potatoes "eyes up" and cover loosely with soil. Do not bury them deep. The sun will warm the soil and soon the eye will grow and roots will form. A little all-purpose fertilizer can be applied when planting, but resist the urge to use too much. Potatoes are not all that picky and not heavy feeders when growing. Your first year of planting, don't use any fertilizer and see what happens. Often gardeners are surprised by how well potatoes perform with no fertilizer when other plants, such as tomatoes, need lots.

Hilling

When the potatoes have emerged and leaves start to show, loosen the soil along one side of the row and pile dirt on top of the newly emerged potato plant. Don't be gentle, just bury the whole plant. Even if it breaks, it will quickly regrow. In a couple weeks, the plant will have grown out of this first hilling and you should do the same, from the other side of the row. On each hilling, bury all visible leaves with about 6 inches of loose soil. Potatoes should be hilled in this fashion until the hills are 12-18 inches in depth. The more time you spend hilling; the more potatoes you will harvest. Potatoes need lots of room to grow in their underground rows. A big hill lets the potatoes grow to their full potential without crowding.

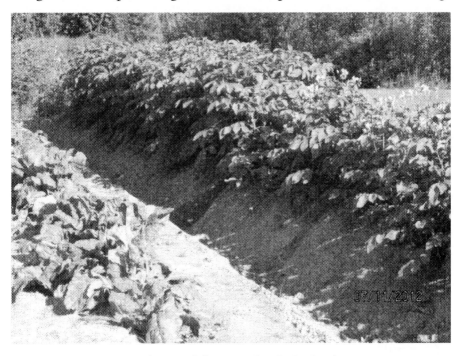

Tim's Mounded Potatoes (Author's Photo)

Caring

Caring for a crop of potatoes means watching for pests, watering if needed, and keeping the weeds at bay. Potatoes are troubled by different pests in different areas. If you see signs of wilting or see bugs all over your potatoes, consult a local garden center and ask for an organic solution. Often insects can be controlled by spraying with soapy water or simply picking the bugs off by hand and squishing (or feeding to the chickens!). The Colorado Potato Beetle is particularly troubling, but easily controlled by organic means.

Potatoes do not need watering as often as other garden vegetables, in fact, over-watering is a bigger concern. Weeds are not generally problematic either as the foliage tends to out-compete most weeds and the hilling process removes those growing alongside the rows.

If I've made it seem as if growing potatoes is easy…it is. They really require very little attention during the growing season. The flowers even look good in a vase!

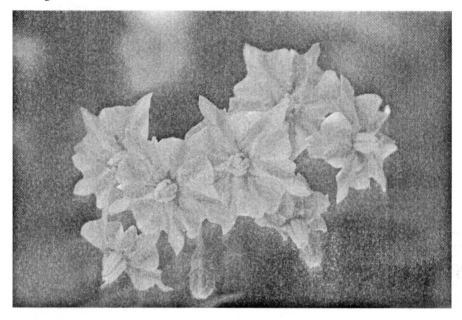

"Potato Flowers" (Pixabay.com)

Harvesting

Once the flowers have started to die off, check for the presence of "new" potatoes. These small golf ball sized tubers are very tasty and can make a perfect "potato hack" meal.

Towards the end of summer, all of the leaves will start to die. This signals the time to dig your potato crop. Often folks will wait until after the first frost for the chore. There are special "spud forks" for digging potatoes or you can get on your knees and simply claw them from the ground.

Be careful, whatever tool you use, to not damage the potatoes as you dig them. Go slow and pile the potatoes between the rows to air dry for a day or two if it's not freezing at night. Otherwise, bring them inside and spread the freshly dug potatoes on the garage floor or other protected area. When first dug, the skins have not formed and the potatoes are susceptible to damage. After thoroughly dried, or "cured," the potatoes develop a thick skin. This thick skin will preserve the potato for up to a year when stored properly.

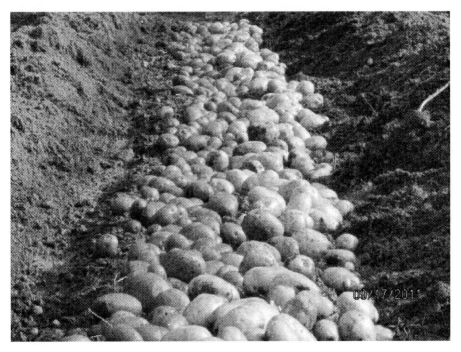

Tim's Harvest (Author's Photo)

Storage

Ideally, potatoes should be stored in a dark, well-ventilated place that is temperature-controlled to 45-50 degrees F and kept at 90% relative humidity. Most people do not have such a place, but most people can find a quiet spot in the corner of a garage or basement where potatoes can be stored for several months. Picked in late September, you can expect to be eating potatoes well past Christmas.

Place the potatoes in old milk crates, burlap sacks, or cardboard boxes. As long as the temperature is kept below 60 degrees and they are kept dark, you should have good success. Root cellars are designed specifically for storing potatoes. If you are not convinced, check with the local garden centers or Cooperative Extension Services for tips for storing potatoes where you live.

However you end up storing your bounty, keep an eye on them for signs of mice. Mice love potatoes. Also watch for mold which indicates improperly stored potatoes. Periodically look through the potatoes and remove any that have rotted as these will spoil the others. After a couple months, your potatoes will do what organic potatoes all do—start to grow.

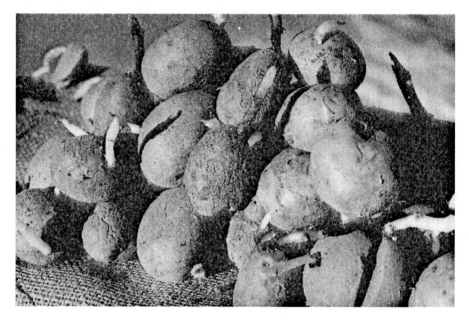

Ready for Spring! (Author's Photo)

At first you'll notice small eyes appearing on your potatoes. When these eyes are 2-4" long, you can rub them off. They will re-grow, but by removing them, you'll extend the time they stay edible in storage. If you allow the eyes to grow, they suck moisture out of the potato which quickly shrivel and dry out. You can successfully remove eyes and sprouts 3 or 4 times before nature wins out and the potatoes are unfit to eat. If you are lucky, your potatoes will last in storage until Spring planting time.

If you managed to extend your storage until the next season, simply plant the potatoes in the garden and watch them grow. Large potatoes can even be cut into quarters as long as each section has an eye or two on it.

Happy growing!

POTATO QUOTES

"I bought a big bag of potatoes and it's growing eyes like crazy. Other foods rot. Potatoes want to see."

- Bill Callahan, American Author

Notes:

Acknowledgements

Thanks to all the blog readers and friends who helped proof-read and provide inputs for content. This book is for you!

A huge thanks to award-winning photographer, and my favorite aunt, Ann Overhulse, of Napoleon, Ohio for the cover photo and potato pictures throughout, and to Brooke H. for being such a great "cover model."

And a special thanks to my wife, Jackie, for putting up with me as I spend more time at the computer than I really should.

And to Mom and Dad for making me eat my potatoes.

About the Author

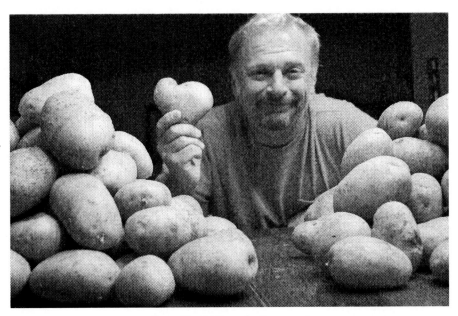

Some Potato Love for Everyone!

Tim Steele and his wife Jackie live in North Pole, Alaska. He retired from the US Air Force in 2004 after 21 years of service and now works in the health care industry, specializing in hospital electrical technology. Tim is pursuing a Master's degree in biotechnology through the University of Maryland. Tim enjoys gardening and tending to his chickens and bees.